PROTOCOLS FOR HEALTH CARE
EXECUTIVE BEHAVIOR

AMERICAN COLLEGE OF HEALTHCARE EXECUTIVES MANAGEMENT SERIES

Anthony R. Kovner, Series Editor

Carson F. Dye

Protocols for Health Care Executive Behavior

A Factor for Success

MANAGEMENT SERIES
American College of Healthcare Executives

97 96 95 94 93   5 4 3 2 1

Library of Congress Cataloging-in-Publication Data

Dye, Carson F.
  Protocols for health care executive behavior : a factor for success / Carson F. Dye
        p.   cm. — (Management series / American College of Healthcare Executives)
    ISBN 1-56793-000-X (hardbound : acid-free)
    1. Health services administrators—Conduct of life.   2. Business etiquette.
I. Title.   II. Series: Management series (Ann Arbor, Mich.)
RA971.D94   1993   362.1′068′4—dc20   93-14057

The paper used in this publication meets the minimum requirements of American National Standard for Information Sciences—Permanence of Paper for Printed Library Materials, ANSI Z39.48-1984. ∞™

Health Administration Press
A division of the Foundation of the
   American College of Healthcare Executives
1021 East Huron Street
Ann Arbor, Michigan 48104-9990
(313) 764-1380

For my family, who have always
given me great love and support:

my parents, John and Evelyn Dye;
a special aunt, Martha Stemple;
my wife, Joaquina, and
daughters, Carly, Emily,
Liesl, and Blakely.

CONTENTS

Part III   Serving the Organization

FOREWORD

I suspect that if readers are embarking on a career in health care management, they might feel that the world they are about to enter contains many ambiguities. Everything can be couched in "maybes," and the decision-making process that they are eagerly looking forward to has been compromised from the start.

However, a reader who is well along in a career in health care management might categorize the feeling as being one of "I've been there before." Reading this book will be a nostalgic trip backward through almost every career situation and experience he or she has had.

The author has attempted to give us a sense of the modern-day health care organization and the relationships that allow it to work successfully. The so-called unwritten rules that govern behavior among individuals are particularly relevant for health care because of the diverse backgrounds and interests of those who work in it. The large concentration of personnel in high-tension situations, in a personal service business where "almost" is not good enough, is ready-made for continued refinement of the working relationship. The focus of the hospital and all of its resources is the care and treatment of the sick and injured. The team effort to accomplish this is steeped in the potential for interpersonal and professional conflict.

This book is rich with examples of this day-to-day "discussion" among people who are committed to the primary goal of patient care but who may be distracted by the turmoil of secondary and opposing aims.

The author is a good storyteller with an excellent "sense of the appropriate." His protocols ring clear, true, and sure as examples of the extraordinary complexity of health care management.

This book serves as a reminder that although in general there is not much new under the sun in management theory and practice, health care delivery in institutions is peculiar and there is much in our history that does not have to be repeated. This book is easy to read, enjoyable, and will make readers nod and think, "I've been there."

Bernard J. Lachner
Retired Vice Chairman and
   Chief Executive Officer
Evanston Hospital Corporation
Evanston, Illinois

PREFACE

Protocols for Health Care Executive Behavior articulates issues that have interested me throughout my 20 years in health care administration. Some executives simply do not possess a "sense of the appropriate." Their personal behaviors offend many, and yet they themselves are often totally unaware of how others perceive them. Few people feel comfortable offering others constructive criticism, and the bad habits and improper conduct continue. Many executives judge their personal success solely by organizational factors such as financial profitability or market share. They rarely reflect upon the effect of their day-to-day behavior and idiosyncrasies. Over the past decade of turbulent times in health care, I have seen and heard about executives who have lost stature within their organizations or even their jobs as the result of inappropriate behavior.

Executives and those who aspire to be executives need to have a "mirror" to help them to reflect upon their actions and how they affect others. This book does not present management principles; instead, it presents the so-called unwritten rules that govern executive behavior in health care organizations. Although, of course, there are many instances in which the right and wrong ways to act are obvious, there are perhaps an even greater number of instances that are "gray"; that is, the right and wrong behaviors are not quite as evident. How we respond over time to these "gray" situations will often determine our personal success or failure.

This book is meant to encourage health care executives to take a closer look at themselves and their behavior, and perhaps change some behaviors and thus become more confident and effective leaders. The concept of protocols suggests that we all often have to "keep a stiff upper lip" and behave at times in ways that hide our true feelings. However, I hope that it is also apparent that a strong value system will make many appropriate behaviors come naturally.

My passion for the subject of this book grew from my amazement at the number of colleagues who have discussed the ideas presented in this book with me and have strongly reinforced my thoughts. We have lamented the fact that graduate programs do not emphasize appropriate behavior and that few seminars ever address the topic. Of course, there are books on personal and business etiquette, and while these are helpful, they are not geared specifically to health care executives and organizations. Also, many of the topics discussed in this book are difficult and sensitive, and it is natural for people to be defensive when something so personal as behavior is discussed. I hope that this book will help to open up discussion on the topic of appropriate behavior for health care executives so that all of us can become more effective leaders.

ACKNOWLEDGMENTS

There are so many people to thank for help with this book. Some helped directly with input and suggestions, whereas others provided me the opportunity to observe their behavior and practice of the "appropriate." First, I thank my wife, Joaquina, my real editor, for great criticism and continual support. My daughters, Carly, Emily, Liesl, and Blakely, were kind and understanding about sacrificing their time with me as I completed the project. I will never be able to repay the support and guidance of my close friend and colleague Steve Strasser, who has taught me so much. Without him *Protocols* would not be. I am also indebted to Ed. Kobrinski, my editor at Health Administration Press, who held my hand, took me into uncharted waters, and challenged the depth of my thinking. Amanda Watlington was especially helpful in supplying needed polish and refinement.

There were many who "led the way" and modeled appropriate behavior for me to observe. The late Dr. Ed Arlinghaus of Xavier University gave me the seeds of thought that started this project years ago. Thanks, Ed—I hope you are watching. Several strong leaders helped me in this endeavor as well as in my career by exhibiting exemplary executive behavior. Thanks must go to Darryl R. Lippman, possibly the originator of the phrase "a sense of the appropriate," and possibly the most "common-sense" executive I know. Others who have demonstrated exemplary leadership in the area of protocols include Michael H. Covert, Donald A. Cramp, William A. Sanger, Lonnie M. Wright, Dr. Edward J. Pike (who helped me better understand physicians), Sister Mary George Boklage, R.S.M., Thomas J. Ruthemeyer, and Michael J. Gilligan. My good friend Mark D. Hannahan was a constant source of support and enthusiasm as well as another excellent role model. Many others who are too numerous to mention reported anecdotes and examples of protocol violations.

I am grateful to those who read various versions and provided suggestions, especially Michael D. Caver, Gretchen Patton, Barbara Mauntler, Carol Thomas, Walter McLarty, Kam Sigafoos, Althea Seagraves, and Mike Scott.

INTRODUCTION

Bosses—especially senior ones—overestimate the significance of their routine decision-making and underestimate the impact of their personal behavior.

Walter F. Ulmer, Jr.

What is implied by executive success? How is it measured or determined? What contributes to the success of senior managers and executives who are recognized as being at the top of their field?

Generally, executives are deemed to be personally responsible for successful organizations. Successful organizations generally have strong financial bottom lines, excellent reputations within their communities, high-quality and loyal medical staffs, and substantial market share. Are the executives really personally responsible for these organizational hallmarks? In many cases, they are. It is the personal leadership skill of many excellent executives that makes their organizations successful.

Successful executives have numerous skills and attributes that contribute to their success. This book will address in detail one of the most important of these—the executive's "sense of the appropriate." Skilled executives and senior managers understand the importance of appropriate personal behavior and relationships and the negative effect that offensive, peculiar, or eccentric behavior can have upon their achievements. They practice "executive etiquette." Most successful executives are aware of their own personality and behavior quirks and work hard at preventing them from undermining their "sense of the appropriate."

Of course, it is possible for executives to exhibit very annoying or offensive habits and behavior and still be successful, as measured by traditional organizational gauges. However, such executives are in the minority; it is rare to find successful executives who are not accomplished at understanding their own behavior and controlling it in a socially (and institutionally) acceptable fashion.

Unfortunately, there are no established codes of conduct that govern all of the various behavioral expectations of business situations. No rules or standards can cover every possible situation executives encounter. However, our society does have certain principles that determine "socially acceptable behavior." Some of these are very clear but, unfortunately, others are not. Senior managers and executives should be aware of these societal principles and the need to follow them. Many of these principles will be presented in this book.

This book does not purport to set forth appropriate behavior protocols for every situation that senior managers will confront. The reader will always have to exercise judgment and keep a sense of perspective when confronted with issues and situations in the workplace. It is hoped that the discussions in this book may serve as a "mirror" to help readers reflect upon and gain a better understanding of their behavior. This book is an appeal to all health care leaders to realize that a "sense of the appropriate" is a very important element of successful management and leadership.

Readers will undoubtedly say many times, "This is merely good common sense." Some will think, "I already know this—why am I reading this?" Others may put the book down after thinking, "This is really simple material—I do not need to continue reading." Some seasoned executives may remain aloof from and untouched by the book's messages. Others may believe that the messages are too conceptual and philosophical to be practical.

However, a large number of executives have read the manuscript and reinforced the concepts behind it. They have shared many "war stories," some of which are used as examples in the book. The fact is that a number of health care executives have had less-than-successful tenures within their organizations because they had a poor understanding of the need for appropriate behavior or were unwilling to change behavior. Some have even lost their jobs because of this.

Within the health care world, the term *protocol* has a rich and deep meaning. It typically refers to the commonly accepted way of doing things to and for patients. The protocol is the right way. The protocol is the way most professionals do things. Many medical protocols are not written in any codified manner. They are frequently passed on from one generation of physicians to another, often during medical rounds. It is hoped that this book can serve as a kind of administrative grand rounds that will help the reader comprehend the significance of appropriate executive behavior. The intent is to help the reader develop a "sense of the appropriate."

The director of one of the leading graduate programs in health administration received a phone call one Monday morning from one of his star alumni who had graduated three years earlier. In those days (early 1970s), an MHA graduate typically entered a health care organization as an assistant administrator and could expect a relatively rapid move up the hospital corporate ladder.

This former student was on the fast track at his first hospital, where he was an assistant administrator, and was about to be promoted to the number-two position under the top administrator. On the morning of his call to the graduate program director, though, he had been asked by his chief executive officer to find another job. It seems that the assistant administrator had attended a medical staff party on Saturday night at the home of the president of the medical staff. He had a few too many drinks and began telling offensive jokes and insulting the other guests.

The formerly up-and-coming young executive was told by the chief executive officer that his behavior had greatly embarrassed the medical staff president and that several other physicians had expressed disapproval. Thus, the CEO continued, the young man's credibility had been damaged and it was unlikely that he could be successful at that institution. He was given six months to find another job.

After he hung up the phone, the graduate program chief reflected upon the performance and behavior of this alumnus while he was in school. He recalled that on many occasions the rest of the graduate class talked of this student's "weekend drunks" and how he loved to "party." He realized that even then there were warning signs of what might occur in the future. Although this young man was an excellent student and had good interpersonal skills on a day-to-day basis, his one shortcoming cost him greatly.

The chair of the graduate program wishes to this day that he had heeded the warning signals and intervened with this unfortunate individual while he was still in school. Perhaps he could have helped him to avoid this humiliating and damaging experience.

In another case, an unmarried CEO with all of the managerial tickets was running his organization quite successfully. After a few years he began dating the ex-wife of a former hospital board member. Although they were open about their relationship, the ex-husband became incensed by it and led a movement to replace the CEO. The ensuing struggle split the board of directors and the medical staff and harmed the hospital for a number of years. The CEO eventually left the organization because of his inability to handle the controversy.

In yet another example, a vice president of professional services was twice passed over for promotion to a COO position. The reason was simple—

several members of the medical staff had petitioned the CEO, indicating that they felt that his past personal relationships with several of the nurse managers would harm his effectiveness. Although the medical staff was comfortable with him in the professional services role, they did not want to see him move higher into the COO position.

These are just a few examples of how managers and executives can lose their effectiveness or, worse yet, their positions because of inappropriate behavior. Executive search consultants relate many stories of senior-level candidates who are technically proficient and have great careers but find their progress interrupted because of some seemingly minor instances of inappropriate behavior or some slight personal idiosyncrasies.

Readers should keep an open mind as they move through this book. They should not be too quick to say "that's not me." Rather, they should use the book to help motivate them to strive to discover character flaws and idiosyncrasies that might seriously undermine their effectiveness as executives and their professional success. Without constant vigilance and self-awareness, it is all too easy to forget one's "sense of the appropriate." Many of the descriptions of problem behavior found in this book can fit many of us, at one time or another.

How This Book Is Divided

This book is divided into three sections. Part I, "Managing Yourself: Self-Discipline," introduces the concept of protocols. It provides a model for executive success that forms the nucleus of the concept of appropriate executive behavior. The principle that character and values drive behavior and that they can be the underlying foundations for the practice of appropriate behavior is introduced.

Part II, "Serving Others," sets forth a number of principles about how executives should interact with others. Implicit throughout is the belief that a new form of leadership, that of "servant leadership," can actually become a strong pathway to personal success.

Part III, "Serving the Organization," provides some insight into the various ways in which executive behavior can be important within the context of the larger organization. Of particular importance are the chapters that address protocols relating to cultural diversity and men and women in the workplace.

Of course, as was pointed out earlier, this book cannot cover every situation that health care executives may encounter. However, the examples provided should help acquaint readers with the basic principles of appropriate executive behavior and how they apply in actual practice.

PART I

MANAGING YOURSELF: SELF-DISCIPLINE

1

Protocols and Executive Success: The Fourth Factor

One thing is certain about the 1990's—there will be numerous changes in the workplace. As companies restructure and downsize, some industries will contract while others expand. As the competition becomes fiercer, getting or keeping a job, or being promoted, will hinge not only on how qualified you are—for there are hundreds of others with similar qualifications—but how appropriately you behave, and how much you look and act the part for that particular position.

Jan Yager, *Business Protocol: How to Survive and Succeed in Business*

Make or Break Behavior

The use or lack of appropriate behaviors or protocols frequently can make or break the careers of individuals in senior-level positions. Senior managers and executives may have superb technical knowledge and excellent administrative skills, be very competent in human resources management, and yet fail in the eyes of others because they lack a "sense of the appropriate." Senior managers and executives may even find themselves out of a job because of inappropriate behavior.

For too long, health care executives have measured success solely along organizational lines. They use such criteria as strong financial bottom lines, increased market share, and positive medical staff loyalty to determine executive success and effectiveness and overlook the importance of appropriate personal behavior. There are frequent seminars and workshops on health care financial management, quality improvement, and strategic planning and marketing. The American College of Healthcare Executives' seminar series provides an ample supply of programs that help senior managers and executives learn how to be more successful. However, by considering only technical or administrative factors, many executive development programs fail to emphasize the very important area of personal factors, which also affect executive success. Although some recent management literature has begun to focus on "leadership" or personal charisma, issues of character or appropriate behavior have not had serious attention.

Letitia Baldrige, a renowned author and expert on etiquette, stated in an interview, "There are a lot of well-educated people in the white-collar world who are very smart about spreadsheets but don't know how to treat other people. And this isn't a matter of their not conforming to some pristine code of etiquette, but simply their having a frame of mind that is selfish and thoughtless."[1]

The focus of this book is not only executive etiquette but also the entire range of senior manager and executive behaviors. It includes taking charge, understanding and working with physicians and board members, and how to work with search firms. Etiquette is important; however, many other professional behaviors and actions must be added to this. For successful executives these are "second nature." Much of their success is how they interact with others, their professional style and grace, their sensitivity to the perceptions of others (and all others regardless of their power and status), and their willingness to modify their own behavior and actions when necessary.

The Four-Factor Formula

The following formula governs this book:

Executive Success =

Effective Technical Skills and Knowledge ×

Administrative Skills and Knowledge ×

Human Resources Skills and Knowledge ×

Appropriate Executive Behavior ("Protocols")

Note that the formula is a multiplicative function with four factors; a zero in any of the factors results in a zero product—zero executive success. To be successful, the executive must have adequate skills in every area. This book focuses on the fourth factor, appropriate behavior.

Throughout the book appropriate executive behavior is referred to as "protocols." In health care, protocols carry a significant meaning. *Webster's* definition of "protocol" closely fits the spirit and intent of this book—a code prescribing strict adherence to correct etiquette and precedence.

Although this book is not a commentary on general etiquette, many protocols do involve the practice of socially prescribed courtesies. Many other protocols, however, suggest character-guided behavior. Character is that element in every person that helps to guide external behavior. Often, external behaviors must be practiced over and over to become "second nature." In some respects, this involves the development of character. Although many parts of this book focus on seemingly simple or obvious behaviors, by practicing them repeatedly the executive can develop a greater respect for others, a true commitment to goals of worthy organizations, and, ultimately, greater personal successes.

What Makes Executives Successful?

As was discussed earlier, successful executives and senior managers require competency in four different spheres:

- Technical skills and knowledge
- Administrative skills and knowledge
- Human resources skills and knowledge
- Appropriate executive behavior (protocols)

The lack of or weakness in any one of these four factors will minimize executive success, whereas strength in these areas will enhance success. The following sections will discuss these factors as they apply to different types and levels of health care executives.

Technical Skills and Knowledge

Most health care CEOs have some knowledge of clinical issues and experience working with physicians. They also have specific knowledge of the legalities of corporations and organizational structures, know how to work with boards of trustees, and understand the importance of public relations and communications and its effect upon their organization. Finally, they have an excellent sense of how the many departments and units of their institutions fit together.

Senior managers and executives know appropriate methods of communication and understand how to coordinate the organization's many daily activities. They are able to assess the performance of their organizations and take steps to improve deficiencies. They also understand the overall role of senior executives and how they fit into the corporation.

Financial executives have specialized knowledge about budgeting, accounting, and reimbursement. Many are certified public accountants (CPAs) and have an in-depth technical knowledge of financial management.

Senior nursing executives have technical knowledge about the professional practice of nursing. Strong senior nursing managers also fully understand the technicalities of nursing care plans and clinical measures of performance. They are aware of particular accreditation requirements of the Joint Commission on the Accreditation of Healthcare Organizations (JCAHO).

Chief human resources officers must know labor and employment law. They also must have specific expertise in benefits and compensation and must understand the technical aspects of human resources information systems and job evaluation programs.

Administrative Skills and Knowledge

Senior managers and executives in all areas and at all levels must be excellent administrators. They must be able to forecast, budget, and plan and know how to coordinate and schedule activities. It is very helpful to have some knowledge of office management. Finally, successful executives know how to run meetings and set strategic planning objectives.

Human Resources Skills and Knowledge

Senior managers and executives must know basic principles of human behavior. They must be able to relate to groups of employees, know how to delegate, and be able to create and sustain a motivating environment. Successful senior leaders have a good grasp of principles of organizational behavior, such as appraisal and feedback and group dynamics. They must also be skilled at conflict resolution and management. Finally, in today's environment stress management (both personal and within the organization) is an important skill for senior managers.

Appropriate Managerial Behavior (Protocols)

This fourth factor is seldom considered in discussions of executive success and is infrequently addressed in graduate school, textbooks, or managerial seminars. Often, however, it becomes the crucial factor for executive success during periods of organizational stress and crisis.

Feedback at the Top Is Impersonal

Unfortunately, the higher managers move in an organization, the less likely they are to hear direct, pertinent, and helpful criticism. The phrase "it is lonely at the top" means more than just that there are fewer people in the same position. There are no peers to provide constructive criticism, nor are there many subordinates who are comfortable providing feedback to a higher-level manager. For senior managers and executives, it is difficult to get any feedback at all on personal issues and behavior. Most feedback relates to organizational issues and does not aid personal development.

In addition, senior executives are in an environment where the only measures that count are statistical or financial. It is the rare vice president who can and will give the president targeted personal criticism. The type of feedback given to presidents and CEOs by their boards is also seldom helpful or specific enough about personal characteristics to help growth.

Other Factors

As was discussed earlier, search firm consultants describe many examples of "successful" executives who had "made it" as measured by statistical and financial indicators and yet found themselves terminated. Some other element apparently cost them their positions. Many times, it is the unquantifiable acts and behaviors that cost them their jobs. These are more than just personality clashes or differences in philosophy or approach. Senior managers should pay closer attention to these seemingly simple and basic proprieties or protocols. Senior managers should try to find their own "mirrors" (others who can provide them feedback) to help them see and reflect upon these issues.

On a daily basis executives encounter numerous situations that require that they respond with appropriate behavior. Senior managers are always being observed by others, ranging from subordinates to board members. Such comments as the following may sound familiar:

From a board member to a search firm consultant who had been secretly called in to begin a search for a new CEO in a medium-sized eastern hospital—"She gets results, but she is really turning off some of the key physicians with her abrasive personality and peculiar attributes. I think that we should begin to look for a new CEO."

From the controller of a small hospital, about his CFO—"We all look busy when he is around—little does he know how we really feel."

From an RN about the COO at a midwestern hospital—"Why didn't she speak to me? She really seems to ignore me when she walks through the hall."

From the majority of executive team members at a leading health care institution about their CEO—"We just don't feel comfortable around him. It is impossible to know what he is thinking, and he is really difficult to read."

From several assistant administrators about a CFO of a large western hospital—"He's a great man to work for as long as you agree with him."

From most of the employees of a religious hospital about their religious administrator—"We've never seen a person whose mood can affect an organization so much."

From a vice president of a medium-sized organization about his COO— "Watch her—she can really turn on you."

From a department head in a well-known medical center about her CEO—"He's just like the waves in the ocean—he'll go away before long and we'll have another CEO."

From a senior executive about a hospital CEO who had extreme mood swings—"He is just not consistent—if he were he would be a better leader."

In none of these cases was any traditional measure of success used to describe these leaders. No one remarked: "Our financial bottom line is not strong enough; I think she will be fired," or "There is too much turnover of senior staff in this organization." For these executives, the functional value of their appropriate behavior was approaching zero, and a perceived zero value in any factor in the success formula results in a zero product in the success formula.

There is more to achieving success than specific organizational measurements. Senior managers and executives should be aware that many of these issues are not covered in courses and seminars. There is no set of generally accepted standards for appropriate behavior, in the way that there are generally accepted accounting principles for financial management. Captain Bligh was an excellent "by-the-book" commander as well as an experienced sailor. Those who have forgotten what happened on the *Bounty* should reread that story.

Note

1. M. Rozek, "Executive Etiquette," *U.S. Air Magazine* (April 1991), 20.

2

GENERAL PROTOCOLS FOR BEHAVIOR

Many protocols for appropriate managerial behavior are applicable to a wide range of situations. The following are broad-based guidelines for behavior in many circumstances that health care executives are likely to find themselves in.

Perception Is More Important than Reality

The following maxim is perhaps the most important lesson senior managers must learn: Management life is the summation of "engineering the perceptions" of other people and helping make their perceptions reality.

Managers who climb high within an organization tend to become distanced from the people around them. As this occurs, they lose sight of what people actually think of them. This distance decreases their ability to assess accurately their actions and decisions. Their reality is not always the reality of those around them. This is particularly true when others increasingly "filter" what they say to senior-level managers. Often, the feedback given to senior managers is inaccurate and is presented too positively. Organization members naturally dislike conveying bad news or disagreement to senior managers. Organizations are full of individuals who are unwilling to become messengers who are killed because of the negative messages they bear.

For example, very few senior executives are openly challenged by employees. Despite the current belief that employees today are more assertive and more likely to challenge authority, most remain relatively quiet. Furthermore, with worsening shortages of health care workers, there are many opportunities for unhappy employees to leave for a new, and perhaps more amenable, organization.

Even when senior executives are challenged or aggressively questioned by an outspoken employee, they will often delegate the handling of the responses to a lower manager. They can escape into the privacy and comfort of the executive suite and remain protected from harsh realities.

The bottom line is that the reality of employees (and often of subordinate managers) is usually not the same reality as that of senior managers. This creates a gap in both parties' knowledge, perceptions, and understanding of the environment. This gap is particularly dangerous for unwary senior managers and executives, for their intentions are often misperceived.

This does not mean that senior managers are always indifferent or insensitive to the needs and difficulties of their subordinates. However, what people perceive is not always what was the intended message. Consider the following:

- If employees from minority groups perceive that senior managers are prejudiced, then their reality is that this is true. To uncover this perception, senior managers must first realize that minority employees have this perception. They then must discover the reason for this perception. The next step is for them to be willing and able to change what is creating the perception.

- If the female secretaries in the executive suite perceive that senior management is a male-dominated enclave and that the environment is sexist, then that is their reality, and it is important for senior managers to recognize, address, and change whatever is causing the perception.

- If a group of subordinate staff members perceives that senior management does not sincerely listen to them and hear what they are really saying, then the reality is that the senior managers are not good listeners. The senior managers should take extra time listening and demonstrate sincerity when staff members discuss concerns with them.

- As senior managers and executives make their rounds within the organization, they need to remember that their staff often perceives that their visit is superficial—and interestingly, often this is true. Executives should take extra time to stop and get to know staff and really listen to their concerns and issues.

Although Tom Peters and Nancy Austin were writing about customer perception in *A Passion for Excellence: The Leadership Difference*, their comments on perception are germane to this discussion. They wrote:

The real problem is that *perception is all there is*. There is no reality as such. There is only perceived reality, the way each of us chooses to perceive a communication, the value of a service, the value of a particular product feature, the quality of a product. The real is what we perceive. As the First Commandment of the formal, written Customer Philosophy at a successful forest-products retailer says: "Feelings *are* facts." Or, in the words of Rothchild Venture's Arch McGill (formerly the youngest vice president in IBM's history): "The individual [customer] perceives service in his or her own terms." (We always add to McGill's line: "... *in his or her own unique, idiosyncratic, human, emotional, end-of-the-day, irrational, erratic terms.*")[1]

What Peters and Austin mean for health care executives is that senior managers should realize what they do, say, teach, or order can be misunderstood because of others' perceptions. Management and leadership involve manipulating frequently misunderstood and misinterpreted words and symbols. Senior managers and executives should make the extra effort, labor in greater detail, and communicate better to ensure that others hear and understand the appropriate, intended messages.

In short, implication does not equal inference. The inference may indeed be very different from the implication.

Many senior managers lose this awareness as they enter the executive suite. Although they may pay lip service to the need to manage perceptions, they often do a poor job of it. Because they are so busy, they often delegate communication to staff people or to lower-level line managers. Their follow-through on issues raised by employees is not as thorough as it may have once been. In their minds, their accountability to subordinate employees decreases as their accountability to higher authority (CEOs and boards of trustees) increases. Consider the following examples:

- The CEO of a hospital in Ohio prided himself on his ability to relate to all levels of employees. He would frequently tell the staff that he used to work in an emergency room and knew what things were like on the "front lines." He believed that he had a lot of credibility with employees and could understand them better than most executives. He would frequently tell his administrative staff that he was a "man of the people."

  In his sixth year at the hospital, there was a serious union organizing drive. During the union campaign, the CEO spent a great deal of time touring the various work areas, talking with employees and encouraging them to support the hospital by voting against the union. After he had toured the hospital to express his support for the prohospital stance, several maintenance employees remarked to the vice president for human resources that this visit to their shops was the first any of them remembered. A number of the housekeeping and dietary employees also observed that the CEO had seldom visited their areas.

The hospital won the election and kept the union out. The "man of the people" once again became busy in the executive suite and seldom ventured out to have any meaningful contact with employees.

- A hospital executive in a medium-sized community was very active in a number of local organizations and service clubs. He believed that his community service was providing excellent visibility for his organization. Yet after his resignation the board committee that was looking for his replacement told the search firm consultant that they wanted candidates who would spend more time on the job and less with the chamber of commerce, Rotary Club, and other activities.

- A well-known executive had held several offices within his state hospital association and eventually was elected president. The following year he was pushed out of his hospital position by his medical staff, who made things very difficult for him. They felt that he had not spent enough time in the hospital and had delegated too much authority to his COO and CFO.

- The CEO of a western hospital made weekly visits to the operating room beginning at 6:30 A.M. to make himself available to the surgeons. He felt that this would enhance his communication with them and show that he was sensitive to their needs and concerns. However, two of the more vocal surgeons told him that they actually viewed his presence as an interruption and a delay. After hearing this, he stopped his early morning visits and met with them at more convenient times.

- Before competition for patients made it uncomfortable for them to work together, two midwestern hospitals had a journal club that held monthly dinner meetings where a member of each senior team presented a report on a journal or book. As the senior staffs of each institution changed and the diagnosis-related group (DRG) era began, the competitiveness between the two hospitals grew.

  One measure of this competition was the increasing elaborateness of the meals served at the club meetings. One of the last of these was an extravagant surf and turf menu. Although the memory of this lasted for but a short time among the executives who enjoyed the feast, the dietary staff of the institution that served it talked about this meal for years to come.

Executive "perks" and symbols create especially strong perceptual messages. The following are especially prone to misinterpretation:

- *Parking spaces.* Senior managers create a negative image when they have reserved parking places, particularly when parking is difficult for other employees. This is not to say that all reserved parking places for senior managers should be eliminated. However, executives should be aware of the negative perception less privileged staff members may have of such highly visible and desirable perks.

- *Executive dining areas.* Consider the negative feelings that elaborate executive dining rooms may create if employees eat in utilitarian cafeterias. The employee cafeteria in one plant in Cincinnati, Ohio, did not even have air-conditioning until the 1980s, but the senior plant management ate in a private dining room complete with linen table cloths and lead crystal.

- *Automobiles.* Without a doubt, an executive's car creates a certain image (more on image building in Chapter 3). The principles in this book encourage senior managers and executives to maintain a professional image. This, however, must be placed in a proper perspective. The CEO who buys an extremely expensive sports car at a time when the hospital is losing money may be sending the wrong message. A CEO in a midwestern hospital bought a new Porsche each year during a time when his institution had several layoffs and reductions in expenses—an especially poor decision in an area of the country where many people work for the U.S. auto industry and "buying American" is viewed as an expression of support for the local economy. Members of the senior management team in a multihospital corporate suite all drove Mercedes Benzes, which created rather negative feelings among the management staffs in the individual hospitals. An executive's choice of automobile should show respect for the regional culture and economy.

- *Catered meals.* Executives who have breakfast or lunch catered to their office several times a week should beware of creating a negative impression for staff employees. There are often very sensible and valid reasons for catered meals (such as private meetings with physicians, significant third party payers, or other business associates). Nevertheless, senior managers should consider the message that free private meals send to other employees. The vice president for human resources in a midwestern hospital was having a celebratory lunch with the employee of the month. The employee remarked that free lunches must be a benefit that came with management jobs. She then asked how many times a week the vice president paid for his own lunch.

- *Laundered shirts.* At one hospital, a private laundry service delivered laundered shirts to male executives. Although the executives paid the full price personally for this service, many employees perceived that the hospital was picking up the tab.

This book deals with the management of perceptions. That perception is more important than reality may ultimately be one of the most important issues for all senior managers and executives. Although perception is *not* reality, it is what managers must work with. Senior managers should be especially cautious of the perceptions they create. This is true whether it involves where they park, how they speak to others (including subordinates), how (or whether) they touch employees, or whether they pay for their own personal postage and stationery.

Show Respect for Other People

Senior health care executives need the support and contributions of many people. It may seem trite to state that human resources are ultimately what make all senior managers and executives successful (or unsuccessful). As many managers move up in their organizations, without realizing it, they may grow less tolerant of others' views and backgrounds and actually show less respect for them. They often have achieved success by promoting *their* ways to the exclusion of other viewpoints. The open exchange of ideas and acceptance of diversity (often including cultural and racial diversity) is not part of the typical executive style, because the executive's career advancement has reinforced his or her own personal views.

Many senior managers achieve their positions by being fiercely competitive and by winning at all costs. Much of the managerial environment involves situations where ideas and plans are presented and then selected in a win-or-lose atmosphere. As this occurs, managers may become somewhat callous toward others. This protocol suggests that senior managers and executives replace callousness with sensitivity to others and respect for their views and practices.

In F. G. Bailey's *Humbuggery and Manipulation: The Art of Leadership* there is a discussion that indicates how managers have lost respect for others. Consider the leadership style exemplified in this description:

> Leadership . . . cannot be done in any honest, open, reasoned, dispassionate, and scientific fashion. The leader must be partisan. He must use rhetoric. He must be ruthless, be ready to subvert values while appearing to support them,

and be clever enough to move the discourse up to a level where opportunism can be successfully hidden behind a screen of sermonizing about the eternal verities. Leadership is a form of cultivating ignorance, of stopping doubts, and stifling questions.[2]

Although all managers may occasionally yield to this mode of leadership, it is frightening to consider this as a recommended style. At some point though, subordinates will see through such deceitfulness. Such leaders will not keep staff and colleagues on their side for long. Furthermore, subordinates working under these conditions are likely to become "yes" people and seldom give their superiors full information. They may hide facts that might cause managers personal or professional discomfort. As a result, senior managers who practice this leadership style may find themselves making decisions without an opportunity to thoroughly examine all the facts surrounding the issues.

Showing respect for others does not mean that senior managers must always capitulate to the others' views or to their methods of approaching issues and problems. It does mean, however, that senior managers must give some consideration to those who have a different approach and show some regard for their beliefs and principles.

Senior managers who are building teams should note that strong teams are not composed of people who all think and act alike. The strongest teams (whether in sports or in management) have team members with different strengths who can play different roles. There is an unfortunate tendency in American health care to select senior team members on the basis of which graduate school they attended or the kinds of organizations in which they have worked. For example, many managers of large hospitals do not believe that managers of smaller hospitals can be successful in large organizations. Executives of teaching hospitals often choose staff only from other teaching hospitals. This "club" mentality makes it hard to develop true respect for others. Although homogeneous groups who attended the same graduate schools or who have worked at similar institutions may have some diversity, they may lack sufficient variety and versatility to develop group strength for optimal team effectiveness.

Over the past several years in this country there has been an increasing awareness and understanding of diverse views, practices, and people. Our society has evolved toward the acceptance of disparate philosophies and customs—of cultural diversity. However, this acceptance has not been fully reflected in the world of the senior management.

This is not to suggest that managers should reject their own values and personal precepts. Rather, it is a statement to encourage awareness that the U.S. work force has become extremely diverse, that this diversity is on the increase, and that this diversity is valuable. There are advantages to the organization when its employees *and* management represent the diversity within the community. As cultural diversity increases, senior managers who have a sincere respect and regard for those who are different from themselves—in age, gender, race, culture, education, and physical and mental abilities—will have an advantage over those who do not.

Get Along with Others

Closely related to the concept of respect for others is the need to get along with others. This critical message will be covered in detail later in the book. Attila-the-Hun managers are a disappearing breed. Senior managers who use the power of their offices and titles to force obedience and team compliance without regard for the need to get along with team members may find it difficult to keep a team together. There are many choices available for high-quality staff members in health care today, and good workers need not stay in oppressive work environments. Despite this, too many senior-level health care managers continue to utilize their power in a negative fashion.

This protocol requires a certain amount of selflessness and a willingness to compromise. It requires sincere listening skills and full group participation in decision making. It also means that the senior executive must occasionally give up the "driver's seat" that he or she has earned and allow others to have a voice in actions and strategies.

More about this topic will be presented in Chapter 7, which deals with interpersonal skills.

Learn to Communicate in
Effective Executive "Sound Bites"

Senior managers and executives usually lead very busy lives. As managers advance in rank and responsibility, the number of activities for which they are accountable increases proportionately. As a result, they have little time to focus on issues and people and few face-to-face encounters with employees. This can become an issue with the employees, who find executives less attentive to their concerns.

Department heads and supervisors clearly spend much more time with their staff than do senior managers. In fact, many first-line supervisors spend the majority of their day with their staff. Senior managers, in contrast, spend very little time with either their subordinate managers or with the employees. Therefore, senior managers must emphasize the quality of the time they spend with employees because of the lack of quantity of time.

Senior managers should view their communication with employees as similar to a politician's sound bites during a political campaign. Unlike lower-level managers, senior executives have only a few moments to communicate and make a favorable impression.

The "sound bite" concept is also applicable to senior managers' communication about work-related matters outside the organization. For example, statements made by executives at civic club meetings or in social situations often are interpreted as being the institution's official stance. Senior managers should carefully monitor what they say in these situations.

The following principles can improve executive sound bites.

Remember That Comments Have Powerful Impacts

Senior managers should carefully calculate the impact of comments they make to staff members and employees during their brief encounters. Comments senior managers may make in passing—for example, while walking to and from the parking garage or during chance meetings in the corridors—are long remembered and often repeated to many other staff members. What senior managers say and how they say it make powerful impressions on employees.

One senior health care administrator prepares several themes and briefly stated strategic objectives that he can talk about during any chance encounters with employees and physicians, or even during meetings where he must make certain impromptu comments.

Carefully Consider What to Say During Meetings

Senior managers and executives should give careful thought to the weight and importance of things they say during meetings. Every sentence and phrase is crucial and is subject to misinterpretation if repeated out of context. Here again the "sound bite" concept is useful. Consider the caution that politicians exercise in campaign speeches. They fully realize the importance of each and every statement.

Maintain an Appropriate Demeanor

Imagine a society in which everyone felt free to express their inner feelings without any inhibitions or obligation to conform to a code of behavior! Most of us would agree that basic courtesy whether sincere or—sometimes—insincere, and a sense of the appropriate are necessities for a civilized society. They also are necessary in organizations.

In order to project an appropriately professional image, executives must sometimes disguise their feelings. This is not to suggest that senior managers and executives should be insincere or phony on a daily basis. However, in the workplace, as in polite society, it is sometimes necessary for executives to conceal their true feelings in order to consistently project a positive and appropriate image.

Professional and appropriate behavior is generally expected of executives, even during times when they may be feeling less than civilized. However, if executives find that they frequently must force themselves to behave appropriately, perhaps they should consider changing jobs. It is not healthy to continually force appropriate behavior. One's external behavior should generally reflect one's genuine inner self, what is commonly referred to as character.

The following situations present some dilemmas about whether to show one's true feelings:

- A guest breaks a piece of antique crystal during a dinner party at your home. Will you become irritated or will you act as though it is really not a problem?

- You and your teenager have a serious argument about grades (or clothes, hair, the car, or one of the many other assorted issues so important to teens) just as you are leaving for work. When you arrive at work, will you leave your angry feelings at the front door or will you allow them to permeate your behavior through the day?

- You work at a university-owned teaching hospital. The college football team has been invited to a holiday bowl game, and you are one of two hospital representatives invited or assigned to go to the festivities. The game is the day after Christmas, which means that you will miss spending Christmas (a very important holiday for your family) with your children and parents. Will you go? If you do, will you be able to act as though you are very glad to be there?

- Your boss has invited you and the other senior executives to a party at his house. The party falls on your spouse's birthday. Will you decline the invitation and tell him why? Will you go? If you go, will your countenance reveal your true feelings?

- On the day of a board meeting at which you are to make a presentation you wake up feeling ill. Will you call in sick and make the presentation at the next board meeting? Will you go to the board meeting, explain that you are ill, and make the presentation as best you can? Will you go to the board meeting, give your presentation, and do your best not to seem ill?

- It is the nicest weekend of the summer and the day of the long-scheduled employee picnic. You, the vice president of operations are expected to attend and stay the entire day—for all three shifts. Your son has asked you to join him and his scouting troop for an overnight camping trip. There is no way you can do both, and you know your son will be very disappointed if you miss the trip. Will you attend the picnic and act very pleased to be there, or will you cancel and join your son? If you attend but cut your attendance short, will you explain why to anyone?

- It is the weekend before Christmas. As the president of your organization, you are expected to attend a number of holiday receptions and parties. You have attended fifteen so far and you and your wife have had no time for shopping or family. This particular Saturday night you are expected at three different parties. Will you go and grin and bear it? Or is there a point at which it is all right to begin to show your true feelings about having to attend so many parties, particularly if you do not like them?

- Your boss has just told you on Friday afternoon that he cannot attend a charity gourmet party that is scheduled for Saturday night. The hospital has bought a table and he wants you to fill in as host. You and your spouse had arranged weeks ago to send the children to the grandparents so that you could enjoy a quiet weekend at home together. You have attended a number of these events and you do not mind them, but your spouse detests them. You really have no choice but to go. Will you go and stay until the very end of the party? Will you act as though you are glad to be there? Will you go late and leave early, making an obligatory but brief appearance? Will you go alone, so that your spouse is spared the ordeal?

- You are the president of your hospital and have for a number of years held open meetings with employees over a period of several days. Because of the size of your organization, you have to hold meetings literally around the clock to accommodate all shifts. This disrupts your sleep patterns greatly, and you are no longer able to adjust to this easily as you did when you were a young assistant administrator. The days spent in the meetings also result in a backlog of work. However, you know that the meetings foster good employee relations and the employees appreciate them. Will you continue these meetings and act happy to be there? Will you decrease the frequency of the meetings? Will you on occasion ask your chief operating officer and your vice president of human resources to fill in for you?

- You have always told employees that they should feel free to come to see you when they have an issue or a concern (as long as they have tried first to resolve it with their immediate supervisor). One employee has been calling your secretary for months, seeking an appointment with you. She has visited with you seven times in the past five months and has never raised a legitimate complaint or issue. She is a very difficult person from whom to disengage, and each meeting takes at least an hour. However, because of her informal influence within the organization, you would prefer not to shut her off. Will you continue to see her and listen half-heartedly, or will you try to persuade her not to continue calling?

The dilemmas in some of these scenarios may have quite obvious answers; others may not. Certainly not all readers would handle them the same way. However, all of the scenarios demonstrate how important it is for executives to maintain an appropriate demeanor, even when they do not feel like it.

Furthermore, it is important for executives to project positive attitudes, because they set the pattern of behavior for the organization. Maintaining and projecting a positive, "can-do" attitude will encourage and inspire employees to do the same. This does not mean that negative information must be distorted (or simply not shared). There is nothing wrong with giving employees honest information—even when it is negative. However, executives should maintain a positive and helpful attitude even (or perhaps especially) when delivering bad news.

To summarize this protocol, senior managers and executives should carefully consider their external behavior and demeanor. On occasion their actions and behavior may have to be different from the way they feel. Successful executives also should monitor their expressions, feelings, and actions so that they appear positive. They should understand that what they say and do can negate the image of competence and professionalism that they want to project.

Put It All on the Table

A successful plant manager at a Fortune 500 corporation was transferred to the company plant with the worst reputation and track record. Not only did this plant have the worst quality record in the company, it also had gone through three wildcat strikes in two years. At a time when other plants producing the same product had seen growth and improved productivity, this plant had experienced a four-year decline.

The new plant manager was greeted and briefed by his senior staff on his first day on the job. The personnel manager told him that she had arranged a meeting with the three local union presidents for the next day. She also told him that the meeting was only a courtesy meeting and that he should not plan to discuss any business at it, and she warned him that the union presidents would probably try to bring up their two leading issues, forced overtime and subcontracting of work. The personnel manager suggested that if they brought these issues up, the new plant manager should tell them that he would discuss them at a later date because he was still getting oriented in his new job.

The three union presidents came into the conference room, and after shaking hands with all three the plant manager said, "Please sit down. I would like to discuss in detail with you now two issues—forced overtime and subcontracting." The personnel manager was stunned, and her amazement grew as the group spent almost four hours discussing the two issues. Within a week, the new plant manager was able to reach a compromise with the unions on these two difficult issues. The union leaders were especially impressed by the new manager's willingness to tackle sticky problems. Within eighteen months, this plant had achieved the highest productivity in the corporation and experienced a total turnaround in labor relations. Not only were there no more wildcat strikes, but during one national strike the local unions actually voted to continue working. One of these local union presidents later became president of the international organization. The former plant manager became the senior vice president of the entire corporation. Working together, they averted a nationwide strike at that corporation. The manager was able to accomplish all of this because of his credibility with the union.

As this example shows, a good manager "puts it all on the table." Whatever the issue or problem, no matter how negative or unsolvable it may seem, even when there is an impasse, it is usually beneficial to put it all on the table and discuss all concerns.

Effective senior managers and executives are problem solvers by nature. However, some senior managers fall into a pattern of simply moving problems around within the organization. They send some issues to a committee, place others on the proverbial "to-do" list but never get to them, and leave still others for the next administration to solve. Many issues are put on hold until a strategic plan is finished or are given to consultants to handle.

Such approaches are not always wrong. Using committees or consultants and buying time for some issues are often viable and appropriate strategies. However, difficulties arise when such strategies become ploys to avoid necessary decision making.

Avoidance of problems is particularly acute in interpersonal relationships. Senior managers may try to avoid certain personal confrontations and will often go to great lengths to postpone meetings or encounters to avoid dealing with interpersonal issues. Many times these clashes can be averted if they are avoided long enough. There may be times when procrastination is the proper approach, but at other times it is totally counterproductive. As a general guideline, procrastination in interpersonal confrontations is appropriate only when a limited cooling off period is needed or when time for fact-finding would help solve the conflict.

The protocol here requires a willingness and ability to face issues that are difficult, touchy, or sensitive. It also requires that senior managers and executives be able to identify matters of conflict or potential conflict. Finally, it requires that senior managers and executives be able to navigate through delicate and sometimes dangerous waters. This requires skill, determination, and courage (more about this later).

To exercise these skills effectively, executives should develop a good sense of timing. They should carefully consider when issues should be brought up and when they should be postponed. Unfortunately, there are no books that provide guidelines in this area. Sensitivity, experience, and observation are the best teachers.

Effective executives are also active listeners. They know and practice good listening skills, they have the ability to listen with understanding and empathy, and they are willing to take the extra time necessary to be an active listener. Communications experts tell us that often people spend most of their time in meetings preparing what *they* are going to say next and thus hear and understand very little of what others say.

Executives should be action-oriented and tenacious in getting problems identified and solved. They should constantly show high energy levels and get others to do the same.

Finally, to be effective problem solvers, senior managers should have courage. Courage in the business world can be derived from several sources, but the most important source is doing one's homework so that one is knowledgeable about the situation at hand. Senior managers and executives should spend time learning *details*. Unfortunately, too many believe that they need only concern themselves with the broad picture and can allow their subordinates to handle the details.

Practice Common Courtesy

The world would be a sad place if people had no manners. It is a sorry commentary that some senior managers seem to have forgotten basic courtesy.

It is interesting to compare how senior managers and executives behave around board members and key physicians with their behavior around less senior or "important" people. There are sometimes unfortunate differences in the level of courtesy. For example, senior-level managers often listen attentively to physicians or board members, but they do not always show the same level of interest in and attention to other employees within the organization.

Executives Should Be on Time

This is an often overlooked courtesy in our society. In fact, the all-too-rare executives who manage their schedules tightly and meet their appointments on time are often called obsessive. Consider how much time is wasted every day as hundreds of people wait outside the offices of senior managers who are running late. Although some may believe that this has become acceptable, it will never be appropriate.

Executives Should Speak Politely

The use of simple courtesy words such as "please" and "thank you" is helpful to any senior manager. Not only is this good manners, but it also shows respect for others. Particularly with employees, these small courtesies will make a positive impression and will often motivate people to give you the results you need.

Executives Should Not Interrupt

Managers must be especially careful not to interrupt others. Often senior managers interrupt others out of impatience and because of their time commitments. However, such behavior is not appropriate, nor is it good manners; and you often lose the opportunity to gain valuable information.

Executives Should Show Courtesy during Presentations

Senior managers and executives should be careful to show courtesy during presentations, particularly when those presentations are made by persons outside of the organization or by those who do not regularly make presentations. If senior managers and executives are visibly bored or obviously are paying little attention to presentations, both within their own organizations and at outside seminars and workshops, they create a very negative impression. Many senior management teams who have become too comfortable with one another fail to show proper attentiveness and are excessively informal even when there are outside visitors.

Six Principles of Business Etiquette

Jan Yager, in *Business Protocol: How to Survive and Succeed in Business*, provides six basic principles of business etiquette that are very relevant to this general protocol:[3]

1. Be on time
2. Be discreet
3. Be courteous, pleasant, and positive
4. Be concerned with others, not just yourself
5. Dress appropriately
6. Use proper written and spoken language

Develop the Art of Concentration

The *ability* to concentrate may be related to intelligence, but the *art* of concentration is related to how one allocates one's time and studies problems and issues. Senior managers and executives often spend their time in the office signing papers, reading and responding to mail, or returning telephone calls. Although these provide momentary feelings of accomplishment and are certainly necessary parts of the job, busy managers should also leave time to plan and to contemplate problems and issues if they are to be truly effective. The following techniques may help accomplish this.

Set Aside Concentration Time

Senior managers and executives should set aside some time each day for thinking, mental preparation, and reflection. They should not use this time for reading. The only acceptable paper would be a blank sheet to write down their thoughts. This time is for reflection and meditation, not for action.

Executives also should try to spend some time each week physically away from the office. One very successful CEO of an eastern hospital slipped away to the medical library on a regular basis to think through issues and problems. In doing this, he found that he could return to the office refreshed and often with new approaches to problems. One CEO of a religious health care organization would return from her annual retreat with a legal pad full of plans and activities and assignments for her senior staff. They frequently joked that they wished she would spend more time praying. The local library might be a good place for creative thinking. Browsing through journals and books one does not normally read, one may find new ideas and approaches.

Busy managers may find it helpful to keep a notepad beside the bed to write down ideas, thoughts, and concerns that come at night. This can help not only one's creativity but also one's sleep.

Learn the Power of Symbols and How to Use Them Appropriately

Symbols are a very important communication mode and have a great deal of significance for people. Practically anything—words, body language, dress, an expensive fountain pen, the house or neighborhood in which one lives, the car one drives—can be a symbol. It may not send the same signal to every person, nor will it always send a signal to every person, but it is important to realize its potential for sending signals.

Consider the following symbols and what they might mean:

- A $250,000 salary and a 40 percent bonus
- A large office with an oversize executive mahogany desk
- Short-sleeved shirts and polyester double-knit sports jackets
- A master's degree from the health administration program at a major university
- An MBA degree from a little-known university
- An expensive black sports car
- A 6,000-square-foot home
- An executive boardroom with fine wood paneling and large swivel chairs for 46 people around a gleaming mahogany table
- A boardroom that is off the hospital cafeteria and doubles as a room for Lamaze classes (the pictures and information for the classes stay permanently on the walls)

These and many other symbols evoke certain images and enable us to describe persons, situations, or institutions they may typify. The important point about symbols is this: Symbols are meaningful. They may be misread or misinterpreted, but they do have meaning. Executives who are unaware of the power of symbols may find that they are sending many unintended messages.

Webster offers the best partial definition of the word symbol: ". . . something that stands for or suggests something else by reason of relationship, association, convention, or accidental resemblance; especially a visible sign of something invisible.

It is crucial that senior managers and executives recognize that they work in a world in which symbols often send more signals and messages than oral or written communications.

Summary

This chapter presents some important general protocols for senior managers and executives to consider. The chapter provides a "macro" view of the executive world to help senior managers and executives consider their behavior, which is an integral and important variable in the formula for executive success, from a broad perspective.

Although they are general in nature, these protocols have specific applications to numerous areas of executive life. The remaining chapters in this book attempt to provide a "micro" focus on specific executive behaviors and will address more targeted issues and concerns.

Notes

1. T. Peters and N. Austin, *A Passion for Excellence: The Leadership Difference* (New York: Random House, 1985), 71.
2. F. G. Bailey, *Humbuggery and Manipulation: The Art of Leadership* (Ithaca, NY: Cornell University Press, 1988), 2.
3. J. Yaeger, *Business Protocol: How to Survive and Succeed in Business* (New York: John Wiley & Sons, 1991), 9–14.

3

PERSONAL EXECUTIVE PROTOCOLS

Personal executive protocols are standards of behavior that govern how executives relate to other people. They also address the expectations that others have of executives as individuals. Without close personal assessment, senior managers and executives cannot improve their "sense of the appropriate." This topic recurs throughout the book.

Personal executive protocols fall into five major categories:

1. Personal appearance
2. Social skills, graces, and interactions
3. Professional image
4. The "entourage" (key staff, including the secretary and others who report directly to the executive)
5. Personality

The fifth category, personality, will not be addressed in great detail because of its complexity. Although it certainly plays a major role in day-to-day protocols, it is addressed in ample detail in other books. Other issues relating to personality are contained in Chapter 7, which covers interpersonal relationships.

It is important to note that an executive's personality—especially as it affects how he or she gets along with others—is one of the most important components of executive success or failure.

Personal Appearance

The effect of personal appearance, not only on first impressions but also for the long term, may be more important than many realize. For the executive who encounters many people for rather brief time spans, appearance is often what people most remember about him or her. The personal appearance of senior managers and executives often is not just the *first* impression but often is the *only* impression.

John T. Molloy (in his book *Dress for Success*[1]) and others have exhaustively addressed the topic of executive dress, so the protocols on this topic will be brief. However, brevity should not imply unimportance. Senior managers and executives would be wise to familiarize themselves with Molloy's work.

Select Clothes Carefully

Executives should carefully select their clothing to present the appropriate executive image. In many respects appropriate executive dress is a uniform, with generally accepted standards and components. These vary somewhat according to region of the country, and successful senior managers should take care to dress according to regionally appropriate standards. For example, dress cowboy boots may be appropriate footwear for a male senior manager at a medical center in Laredo, Texas, but would look very out of place on a senior manager in Boston. Navy blue suits may be the uniform of choice for male executives in Chicago hospitals but might seem too formal in a rural area, where executives usually wear sport coats.

Women managers and executives may want to exercise an especially high degree of care and discretion in choosing clothing. Fairly or unfairly, women executives must dress in a manner that ensures that they will be taken seriously as executives. Although women executives certainly need not dress like men, their clothing should, like men's clothing, be conservative and unostentatious. They also should be careful to observe regional conventions for women executives' clothing. For example, a woman's dress might be quite appropriate in a Philadelphia hospital but look very out of place in a rural midwestern hospital.

Appropriate executive attire is not intended to express an executive's individuality. Clothes that are too individualistic, stylish, or contemporary are usually inappropriate. When trying to decide whether an outfit is too extreme, ask whether people are likely to notice the clothing more than the executive. If the answer is yes, the clothing probably is not appropriate executive attire.

Executive attire should, of course, be clean, pressed, and well-fitting. Shoes should be in good repair and freshly shined. Executives should also be sure that their hair and nails are neat and clean and well tended. If beards or mustaches are worn, they should be neatly trimmed. Women executives should avoid elaborate hairstyles, too much makeup, and flamboyant jewelry and accessories. The executive is not just representing himself or herself but also the organization.

For this reason, organizations should consider establishing clearly worded printed guidelines about appropriate work attire. Executives should take care to handle dress code violations professionally and sensitively. If a female employee wears inappropriate clothing a male manager should ask a female manager to discuss appropriate work attire with the person. The reverse should also be true, if the inappropriately attired subordinate is male and the manager is female.

Maintain Good Personal Hygiene

It may surprise some readers that personal hygiene is mentioned at all in a book for health care executives. However, search consultants cite a number of examples in which candidates for senior-level positions had poor personal hygiene that kept them from getting the job. Some candidates had an offensively strong garlic scent on their breath. Several other executives were ruled out because their excessive use of cologne, aftershave, or perfume damaged their executive image. Other candidates were taken out of running because of foul body odor. (This is certainly an area where few senior-level managers can expect direct feedback.)

Avoid Potentially Offensive Personal Habits and Behavior

Smoking, picking one's teeth, chewing gum, poor table manners, and nail biting are just a few personal behaviors that others often find offensive. Senior managers should work hard to avoid these habits and behaviors.

Here again, search consultants cite numerous examples of otherwise competent executive candidates who have had their images impaired by offensive personal habits. One candidate for a vice-presidential position picked his teeth in the presence of the search consultant and the COO. This gauche act cost him the job.

Another candidate for a senior-level position clipped her nails in front of the CEO's secretary while waiting in the reception area for an interview. This did not cost her the position, but it made a very negative impression on the secretary, who mentioned it to the CEO.

A COO of a midwestern hospital tells of a candidate for vice president for business development at a Catholic hospital who pulled up his socks in front of one of the nuns during his interview. The sister felt that if he did not know better than to do that during an interview, he might make other mistakes in judgment and, in her view, was not appropriate for the position.

Although the candidate had the necessary technical experience, he did not get an offer.

In summary, senior managers and executives should remember that their personal appearance and behavior are crucial parts of their executive image. Although few people can look as if they stepped out of a magazine, all of us can be well groomed and project an executive image. Care and attention to personal details reflects positively upon all senior managers and executives.

Social Skills, Graces, and Interactions

Unfortunately, in today's busy, high-pressure workplaces common courtesy and social skills have taken a backseat to seemingly more important issues. Society (including busy executives) often forget to take the little bit of extra time required for common courtesy. However, the appropriate practice of courtesy can offer senior managers and executives an advantage when working with others. As the competition among large numbers of well-qualified candidates increases for health care management positions, good manners, well-developed social graces, and effective interpersonal skills can give a candidate an edge over the others. On the job, health care managers can enhance their leadership effectiveness by exhibiting social skills and graces and basic courtesy. One CEO of an eastern hospital is well known for his excellent manners, social graces, and skillful interactions with others. Those who have worked with him throughout his long, successful career always point out his beautiful manners above all characteristics.

The intense pressure on high-ranking health care executives may lead them at times to forget basic politeness. This mild rudeness is often over-looked or considered insignificant by those who spend a great deal of time with them. As a result, some executives may continue their impolite behavior. However, this type of behavior will definitely be noticed by people who do not work with them often and probably will make a rather negative impression. A first or occasional impression is often a long-lasting one. Habitual discourtesy can be very damaging to one's career.

Show Courtesy to Others

Courtesy actually extends *beyond* outward behavior or actions. Courtesy shows how people see themselves in relation to others and is a good indication of their respect for others. One's level of courtesy also shows how willing one is to be considerate of others and is a measure of one's degree of selfishness.

This does not mean that selfish or rude executives can never be successful—they can. Nor does it mean that respect for others is an absolute criterion for promotion and advancement. However, courtesy and respect for others characterize the majority of successful executives. Executives have a large degree of control over the lives of others. Businesses would be more respected and probably more successful if those in control had a true and sincere sense of respect and consideration for those who work for and with them.

Other than remembering to say "please" and "thank you," what are some guidelines for executive courtesy?

Show extra respect for service employees. Executives should show great respect for those employees who provide basic services. The health care industry has a large number of support service staff, and all senior managers can expect to have contact with people in service positions. Because service employees often are paid less and have less education than executives, they may be looked down upon and denied the respect they deserve. However, wise senior managers will appreciate the value of these workers. Employees who handle basic service jobs such as those in the dietary and housekeeping departments are crucial to the health care organization's operation and deserve true and sincere respect. Because they often relate directly to the public, these employees are of great value to the organization's image.

Practice basic courtesy every day. Senior managers and executives should strive to practice basic courtesy at all times. A group of employees once remarked about a certain CEO whom they respected greatly, "It's the little things that he does that we like. He is so kind and courteous."

Project a positive attitude. Executives should not complain—that is, gripe without proposing a solution—about anything or anyone. They should learn to take problems in stride and concentrate on finding solutions. Targeted comments that identify problems and propose solutions are positive executive behavior. General griping and grumbling is not.

This protocol does not suggest that everything is always "sunshine and blue sky." Executives and managers often must express dissatisfaction with people's performances or undesirable situations. The key issue is *how* the executive expresses dissatisfaction. The object is to resolve the problem, not merely to vent one's dissatisfaction. Express concerns as opportunities rather than problems. View problem-solving challenges as ways to improve service and quality.

One executive of a midwestern hospital had such a positive approach that she would always tell her staff that problems were not problems, they were opportunities for positive change. The longer her subordinates worked with her, the more positive their own attitudes and outlooks became. An extra benefit was that problems were solved quickly and effectively.

Avoid excessive informality. Executives should try to avoid excessive informality. It is wonderful to work with people one likes and respects, but executives and managers should avoid inappropriately familiar remarks or actions, such as the use of nicknames among executives, practical jokes that are taken too far, or horseplay among executives. The most productive work settings are those which have some formality and decorum; such environments are seldom very "laid back."

In addition, executives should avoid sharing personal problems with coworkers. Personal conversations take valuable time away from work and often cause the executive to lose the respect of subordinates.

Avoid moodiness. Senior managers and executives should attempt to maintain an even disposition and outlook and avoid seeming moody. A vice president of nursing in a midwestern hospital once said this about her CEO: "I wish he would either be a son-of-a-gun *all* of the time or be considerate *all* of the time—I would just like some consistency so I would not have to guess what kind of a mood he is in each day."

Another hospital CEO was so moody that her secretary became quite popular because each day she informed others of her boss's mood and advised them about whether or not they should wait for a "better" day to bring issues to her.

Avoid profanity and sarcasm. Profanity is never appropriate in the workplace. Use of profanity may mean that a person is becoming too emotional about an issue and is losing control. Loss of control is not, of course, how senior managers should approach problems. Profanity often is used for effect or emphasis or to "spice up" routine conversations. However, senior managers should find other words and ways to accomplish this. Other workers, both peers and subordinates may be offended by the profanity, even if they do not say so. Profanity can distract from the message and intent of verbal communication.

Sarcasm, too, is out of place in the executive suite. If executives and managers must offer criticism or reprimands, they should not resort to sarcasm, which, like profanity, distracts from the message.

Be an active listener. To improve interactions with others, executives should be sincerely concerned with others' feelings and beliefs. This is best demonstrated and accomplished through active listening. Active listening requires a sincere desire to hear and understand what others are saying, as well as acceptance of their right to their viewpoints. Executives should verbally acknowledge the comments of others and give them the chance to offer additional information about their subject. Without constant demonstration of active and sincere listening, executives will eventually lose credibility and their successes will diminish.

To become better and more active listeners, executives should avoid dominating conversations. If others cannot participate in the exchange, it is not a dialogue, it is a monologue.

Executives should also learn to show concern and empathy when others express concerns or worries but should avoid describing their own personal experiences with similar problems. Senior managers should realize that people often simply want to express themselves and not receive a lesson on how to cope with their difficulty.

One of the most widespread areas of executive weakness is the lack of listening skills. Whether caused by lack of time, inability, or executive egos, it is seemingly present in most management circles. It is hard to convince others that this is a problem—but it is one area where in the experiences of this author, all senior-level managers would do well to closely examine themselves.

Maintain self-control. Senior managers and executives should consider the risks involved if they are unable to maintain self-control, particularly during times of high stress. Losing control may also mean losing the attention of the group being led and may mean that some of the group will look to others for leadership. Society places a high value on remaining calm and composed during a crisis. Successful executives may appropriately show emotion from time to time when trying to inspire, but they should never seem to lose their self-control. Society expects leaders to maintain self-control.

Controlling emotions is especially important for women executives. There is an unfortunate stereotype of women as being more emotional than men and being more likely to lose control in difficult situations.

Learn how to apologize. Executives should become adept at the art of making apologies. Some executives find it difficult to admit mistakes and to apologize whether to peers or to subordinates. However, executives, like all humans, make mistakes, and when they do, a gracious apology is in order. Executives should correct themselves and attempt to make things right with the offended person.

Use "executive manners" outside the workplace. Senior managers should remember to use "executive manners" and courtesy at the golf course, on the tennis court, at the exercise club, even when driving a car. Executives in public places cannot allow themselves to lose control of their temper or act out in other negative ways. Even when not on the job, they are representatives of their management team and their organization and are always "on public display." Improper behavior outside the executive suite can have negative ramifications inside the suite.

Use caution when speaking freely. Senior managers and executives must exercise extreme caution when speaking freely. Because they are privy to confidential and "sensitive" information, and because their ideas and opinions carry a lot of weight, senior executives and managers can "drop their guards" only with those whom they trust implicitly to be discreet. On occasion, senior managers and executives divulge information and bring others into their confidence in order to establish a bond of trust and to encourage others to reciprocate. However, this should be done with caution.

Strengthen relationships by sending notes. A good habit for senior managers to develop is the sending of thank-you and congratulatory notes. Any time someone has done something that helps the organization or has achieved something of merit, a note is in order. Sending such notes is an excellent way to stay in touch with others and to strengthen relationships. Many successful CEOs and other senior managers keep a supply of notecards in their desks and send notes on a frequent basis. Notes of sympathy, although very difficult to write, should be sent when appropriate.

Show Warmth, Caring, and Concern for Others

The ability to show warmth, caring, and concern for others is an important, if not essential, element of executive success. Sincere concern for others and their interests and welfare helps executives avoid developing an ego-centered, overly aggressive professional personality. Although successful executives cannot be meek, they should try to avoid being too pushy. Developing a genuine concern for others can help in this respect. In addition, executives who do not show concern for others may find that others will reciprocate by showing no concern for their interests and welfare. Showing concern for others is not only good manners, it also is an appropriate show of respect for others. Senior executives and managers can demonstrate warmth, caring, and respect for others in many ways, including those discussed below.

Smile! A smile is a simple, everyday thing, but it can be a powerful motivator. Consider how seldom many senior managers smile at others. Often employees believe that senior managers do not care about them because they do not smile at or speak to them. Although senior executives are often preoccupied with serious issues and concerns, they should avoid projecting a lack of concern for employees.

Maintain eye contact. Senior managers and executives should take care to look people in the eye when speaking or listening to them. Eye contact is, in our society, suggestive of sincerity. Increased eye contact creates a perception of truthfulness and sincerity.

One CEO of a health care system will not hire any senior-level person unless that person establishes eye contact early in the initial interview. He believes that eye contact indicates high confidence and the ability to achieve goals. This may or may not be a valid assumption, but it is true that most people believe that eye contact should be maintained by people who are interacting.

Have a sense of humor. Senior managers and executives should have a good sense of humor and be able, on occasion, to laugh at themselves. Many human resources efforts are targeted at bringing employees closer to the organization's senior executives. One of the best ways is for senior managers to maintain their senses of humor and laugh with employees and at themselves. This allows employees to identify more personally with executives.

Be liberal with praise. A number of employee surveys have shown that one of the leading concerns among employees is the lack of day-to-day recognition from senior managers and executives. Formal organizationwide recognition systems are often ineffective at addressing this concern. What employees really want is ongoing acknowledgment and recognition on a day-to-day personal basis. Senior executives and managers can accomplish this by recognizing praiseworthy actions and accomplishments orally or in writing.

Being liberal with praise also applies to those who may not be subordinates. Peers will also appreciate sincere praise; in the highly competitive world of senior management, praise from peers is almost nonexistent. Often peers can be praised for nonspecific accomplishments. For example, one can mention how much one enjoys working with someone. Peer praise can often serve to strengthen personal relationships and enhance team effectiveness.

Avoid "cute" criticism. Executives should avoid giving cute or facetious criticism. Criticism should always be constructive and targeted to specific behavior. When people (particularly peer-level senior managers) are familiar and comfortable with one another, they may tend to make cutting remarks that supposedly are offered in jest (e.g., comments about weight or dress).

However, such "facetious" comments may be taken negatively by the recipient, who may not let on that he or she feels offended. Obviously, this can cause much future harm and should be avoided.

Remember names. Senior managers should pay careful attention to names when meeting people, and make a special effort to remember them. Repeat a person's name when you're introduced for the first time, and write it down later, if necessary. Learning and remembering names are excellent ways of demonstrating care for others.

Building and Maintaining a Professional Image

Jan Yager defines image as "the sum total of our appearance, speech, demeanor, and even our people skills."[2] In this book, a professional image is the positive impression that senior managers want to give others.

In essence, image is a perception and can be either accurate or inaccurate. An image can also be an illusion—something that seems to be there but really is not. This discussion of image building does not advocate insincerity or distorting the truth. Instead it advocates the cultivation of positive attributes and characteristics that will project an overall positive professional image.

Because a senior manager or executive's image is what others see and believe about him or her, its importance cannot be overestimated. The senior manager's professional image helps create his or her leadership environment and signals others about how he or she fits within the organization and what role he or she will play. Thus image both is very personal and very public.

A very successful CEO of a southern hospital, when he is not making strategic and analytical decisions, spends most of his time building, maintaining, and polishing his image. He believes that an important part of his job is to create a certain belief on the part of those around him (employees, physicians, board members) in his abilities and talents. That is what he means by image building. He recognizes that his image is a key part of his leadership style.

One's professional image is built on three foundations and is viewed by seven interest groups or "publics."

The three foundations of professional image are

1. professional ability;
2. achievement through results; and
3. personal characteristics.

Note that the first two relate specifically to one's work image, and the third relates to one's personal image.

Among the various "publics" who perceive this image are employees of the organization as a whole; employees who report to one directly; supervisors and middle managers; physicians; purchasers of services (e.g., third party payers, managed care groups); and the community as a whole.

Thus personal image can be defined as the combination of what is done (foundations) and what is seen (public perceptions).

Developing a Good Work Image

A good work image can be developed and enhanced by developing a strong work ethic, as defined by the practices discussed below.

Arrive early and stay late. Successful executives should arrive at work on time or even early and work a full day or even stay late. The focus here is not on simply *putting in the time* but rather on *putting in the time to get results.* Senior-level positions demand a great deal of time in order to focus on detail and cover the myriad of issues requiring attention. Although effective time management is a crucial skill for all executives, one should be careful to cultivate the image of a hard-working executive who has the right to expect diligent work and punctuality because he or she is diligent, hardworking, and punctual.

Staying focused on priorities. Executives should be meticulous about keeping track of issues and priorities. They should continually evaluate priorities and reassign them when needed. An objective-based work style should become second nature.

One very successful COO of a midwestern hospital keeps track of her objectives and accomplishments by writing down fifteen to twenty objectives for each three-month period and monitoring her progress toward accomplishing those objectives on a weekly basis. At the end of each three-month period she assesses her accomplishments and feels that she has made excellent progress if she has achieved at least three-quarters of the fifteen to twenty objectives. She now asks her department heads to follow the same procedure and holds quarterly team review meetings. At these meetings team members review their progress over the past three months and share their objectives for the coming three months.

Developing a Good Personal Image

Show courtesy and social grace. Many of the issues raised in the earlier discussions of courtesy and social graces aid in the development and maintenance of a positive personal image.

Show attention to and respect for all constituencies. All of the many "publics" with whom senior managers and executives interact should be given consideration and attention. They will not all take the same amount of time and effort, and they do not all have the same potential to affect one's professional success or failure, but all must be given attention and respect.

Many senior managers overlook this protocol and "play to only one section of the theater." For example, they focus only on the medical staff to the exclusion of employees or spend too much time with board members and forget the constituents back at the hospital. Some effective executives actually keep lists of people whom they contact on a regular basis simply to "touch base" and check out their concerns and issues. This is an excellent way to maintain a broad base of support.

Survey all "publics." Senior mangers and executives should constantly survey all of their constituencies, both formally and informally. For example, all members of the medical staff and all employees should be surveyed at least annually about concerns and problems.

Executives should try to understand how the various "publics" in the organization interact with one another. For example, employees or medical staff members who feel that they are not getting anywhere with senior management will often go to board members to seek resolution. Executives should take note of the interrelationships among these groups of people and try to anticipate how they might affect decision making.

Be tenacious. Tenacity is a characteristic that stands out more than any other in building a professional reputation. Effective senior managers know that not all issues will be simple, not all decisions will be clear-cut, and not all mistakes and pitfalls can be avoided. The ability to bounce back and keep coming at the problems is highly prized. If one is tenacious, almost all problems can be overcome. Senior managers who are starting to wither from the pressure of various situations should remember the old adage "this too will pass." Those who show determination and persistence are usually successful.

Most success is built upon what people believe that they can do *in the future* rather than the successes they have had in the past. Consider the teenager who shoots a basketball at a hoop for hours on end. He or she does not keep at it because of great successes on the court in the past but rather because he or she hopes for great success in the future. Tenacious senior managers hold fast to future goals and remain focused upon them in spite of barriers and hassles. Tenacity perhaps more than any other characteristic will create a strong personal image.

Personal image is one dimension of an executive's success. Although not quantifiable, it is an integral part of how one is perceived.

The "Entourage"

Senior managers are the ones who "manage managers." The abilities and skills of the managers who work for executives often reflect directly upon the executives themselves. A CEO of a midwestern hospital who had just praised the strength of her staff in a board meeting was told by the chairman, "Well, that is expected." What was meant, of course, is that successful executives are expected to recruit and manage a successful staff. The sections that follow discuss key members of the executive's "entourage."

Secretaries

In addition to top-flight skills, good secretaries should have excellent manners and should be able to handle interactions with others, whether in person, over the telephone, or in written correspondence, with courtesy and tact. Executives should emphasize to their secretaries the need for courtesy and remind them that the secretary's conduct reflects upon them. The secretary who helps present a positive image for the executive will present a professional image and will enhance his or her boss's professional image.

It is highly desirable for secretaries to maintain neat and orderly work areas. They should have ample storage space so that the desk and the surrounding areas can be kept free from clutter. Bulletin boards and walls should be neat and uncluttered, and outdated notices and memos should be discarded. Personal mementoes should be discreet and kept to a minimum. These suggestions might seem insignificant, but they all contribute to the secretary's—and hence the boss's—professional image and appearance.

Successful and effective secretaries are aware of the powerful impression created by written communication. The documents they produce are free of typos and grammatical errors and follow proper formats and protocols. They keep a good grammar text and dictionary close by for ready reference.

Executives should have frequent meetings with their secretaries to plan strategy and set priorities. Whenever possible, senior managers should include their secretaries in decision making and should explain the philosophies and reasoning behind as many decisions as possible. Without frequent meetings, there is often a great deal of miscommunication and confused expectations. Executives should avoid being so busy that they cannot conduct routine priority-setting sessions.

Subordinate Managers

Executives should share as much information as possible with their key staff members. All too often senior managers keep information from their staff to maintain power; however, the power the team gains from having the information is often more beneficial to the organization and to the senior manager. The more subordinate managers feel in the know about issues within an organization, the more they will feel tied into the team and the more support they will give their boss. They will develop an increased sense of personal loyalty and team solidarity.

One new CEO of a large prestigious health care institution inherited a very strong senior team put together by the previous CEO. The previous CEO had a clear philosophy of sharing all kinds of information with her entire team. The new CEO, however, did not share his predecessor's philosophy. He immediately made it clear that he would be the conduit for all information that flowed to and through the team, he minimized the amount of information sharing among the team members, and he kept much high-level information to himself. Feeling powerless and shut out, all but one member of the previously strong team had moved on to other organizations within a year.

The following principles are especially useful in working with subordinate managers.

Share the management philosophy. Senior managers should be certain that the team knows their management philosophy. They should explain why they made certain decisions and took certain approaches. This will help subordinate managers interpret the decisions and approaches to others. Also, the more subordinate managers know about a senior manager's management philosophy, the better they are able to anticipate his or her responses to many of their questions, and the more likely they are to tailor their requests and actions to fit well with that philosophy.

Stay in touch with key subordinates. One of the biggest complaints of middle managers is that their senior management does not spend enough time communicating with them. They frequently express concern that they have not been informed of certain facts and details that are necessary for the operation of their departments.

Senior managers may find it useful to hold weekly meetings at which every team member relates the key items on his or her weekly calendar. This lets the team know what each member's key issues are for the week and thus enhances teamwork. It also lets the team clarify difficult or sensitive issues on the spot and provides motivation to start the week.

Identify the roles that team members play within a group. Members of any team actually play *two* different roles: their formal role, which is related to their job, and their informal role, which is related to their personality. Consider these two roles when making hiring decisions so that team members complement one another.

The CFO's formal, primary role is financial management; the vice president of human resources' primary role is personnel administration; the vice president of nursing's primary role is overseeing nursing care, and so on. However, the informal, secondary role of each of these team members may be very different. Some of the roles that group members may play include:

- Cheerleader—a group booster who is particularly helpful during times of stress.
- Historian—typically has been with the organization for many years and remembers why everything was done as it was and what is stored behind every door.
- Traditionalist—much like Tevye in *Fiddler on the Roof*, he or she helps the group remember the traditions and heritage that make the organization unique.
- Visionary—keeps an eye on the future and helps the group focus on future goals.
- Planner—helps to formulate goals and visions into practical language and plans that the group can use to move forward.
- Parent—is the mom or dad of the group who provides the often needed guiding influence.
- Implementer—helps to overcome obstacles and get the job done.
- Evaluator—keeps the group focused on how their accomplishments are viewed and contributes to the vision and goals of the group.
- Clarifier—in times of confusion, helps clarify key issues and questions.
- Conscience—keeps the group focused on ethical and appropriate actions, as well as on the special needs of diverse groups within the organization.
- Technician—handles the technical details of group life, including the maintenance of the room temperature, supplying pads and pens, keeping the seats in the meeting room neat, and cleaning up after the group leaves.
- Energizer—has the enthusiasm and energy to get the group excited and energized in approaching their tasks.

- Devil's advocate—by pointing out all the reasons not to do some-thing, he or she helps save the group from the embarrassment and failure of poorly thought-out programs.
- Compromiser—dislikes conflict and helps others find a compromise.
- Quiet follower—uncommon within senior groups, this person is a quiet, passive participant in the group process. Managers should not assume that the quiet follower is an ineffective member of the group. He or she may be uncomfortable speaking out in group settings but may be an efficient implementer of group decisions.

It is often through informal, secondary roles that a team comes together to achieve great goals. Effective executives realize this and develop balanced teams.

Personality

One last area must be considered in looking at the executive's personal protocols—the ability to serve as a role model. Perhaps the best way to inspire, lead, and ultimately succeed is to set an example for others. Many leaders who have been deficient in other areas have made the required personal sacrifices and by setting examples for others have become suc-cessful. Whether or not an executive is able to succeed in this way is largely dependent on his or her personality.

The ability to do what they are asking others to do is the definitive test of successful executives. Such executives show by example that they are able and willing to do the necessary work to get things accomplished. In order to set such an example, senior managers and executives should follow the basic but powerful protocols described below.

Do everything as well as possible. Executives should perform to their fullest in their jobs. Whatever they do should be done with excellence as a goal. Executives should maintain the high level of energy needed to do jobs correctly. They should take the extra time to study details, to prepare a little better than others, or to cover additional ground. Yes, this means making sacrifices—mostly in terms of leisure time—but it is necessary if executives are to serve as effective role models.

Maintain enthusiasm. Senior managers should be as enthusiastic as possible in all that they do. People who are negative or complain frequently about how impossible things are cannot set good examples and do not have the appropriate attitudes to be strong senior managers.

Let work become a passion. Senior managers should approach their work with an intensity and a desire that signal others that they enjoy doing it.

Go above and beyond. Senior managers should do more than just what is expected; they should "go the extra mile." They should be constantly looking for additional ways to contribute to the success of their organizations. This means, at times, volunteering to serve on extra committees and work groups.

Successful executives typically put in long hours. Although the value and wisdom of expecting senior managers to work such long hours is often debated, the fact remains that senior managers frequently are judged by the number of hours they put in.

Avoid excessive perks. Rank should not always have its privileges; executives should beware of taking inappropriate or excessive executive perks. Too many executives have had their reputations permanently ruined because they used their rank and perquisites for personal gain. Although health care executives are not as much in the public eye as are politicians, they too need to stay "squeaky clean" and avoid even the appearance of impropriety. The personal use of company property, padding expense accounts, or having excessive executive benefits or pay programs are just a few examples of inappropriate use of rank toward one's personal advantage.

Be aware of regional and geographic variations. When considering any of the protocols suggested in this chapter or anywhere within this book, readers must always take into consideration regional variations in customs and courtesies. What is considered appropriate behavior will differ from one area of the country to another. This is particularly true with regard to personal appearance and certain day-to-day courtesies and social graces. Although the differences are too many to enumerate here, they are nonetheless important. The best guideline to use in most situations is simple: "When in Rome, do as the Romans do."

Summary

This chapter on personal executive protocols is very important because it deals with enhancing executive effectiveness. However, it also deals with a topic that can be controversial. People typically resent being told to fit into the same mold as others, and directed as to how to dress and act. Yet, the importance of their "conformity" is the basic premise of this book. Social protocols—socially correct and appropriate behaviors—have existed as long as people have gathered together in social groups. Although some differences and creative self-expressions are at times suitable, some set order and consistency are necessary to preserve order, enhance predictability of behavior, and to avoid disorder and confusion.

Senior managers should closely examine their actions and behavior, which speak much more loudly than their intentions and their words. The best place to start such self-examination is with a careful analysis of their conduct and deportment.

Notes

1. J. T. Molloy, *Dress for Success* (New York: P. H. Wyden, 1975).
2. J. Yager, *Business Protocol: How to Survive and Succeed in Business* (New York: John Wiley & Sons, 1991), 18.

4

EXECUTIVE VALUE SYSTEMS: THE FOUNDATION FOR PROTOCOLS

The word *character* is used to describe a person's essence or personality. In ancient times it referred to a mark that was scratched permanently on something in order to identify it. *Character* in this book refers to a person's true inner being. *Character* can also mean high moral quality or wholesomeness.

Protocols describe appropriate external behaviors, but they do not address internal, causative factors. In an ideal world, senior managers and executives would behave appropriately because such behavior is the natural expression of their inner selves; the protocols are instinctive and intuitive. In the real world, however, most executives follow protocols for demeanor and conduct because they know them to be appropriate, even if they do not always "come naturally." However, the constant practice of appropriate behavior helps to build character so that appropriate behavior becomes natural and instinctive. The following are key assumptions that apply to "character building."

1. The desire to develop genuine (as contrasted to compelled) appropriate responses to others is the hallmark of positive leadership in that appropriate behavior does not have to be forced.

2. Repeated practice of appropriate executive behavior will over time build character and foster continued growth and development.

3. As their characters becomes more upright and worthy, senior managers and executives will become better role models and mentors.

Values and value systems are the foundation for behavior and character. The values of senior managers and executives are important factors in how they behave.

Values are those principles that people hold on a long-term basis, deep-seated beliefs that usually do not change over time. Values in many respects serve as standards that guide behavior. Values differ from attitudes in that attitudes tend to be short term, to represent feelings and opinions about specific issues and problems, and to be much more numerous than values. Values embody longstanding views and convictions about more "global" matters. Values guide attitudes and direct decision making. Value systems, the sum total of a person's individual values, are already fully developed by the time people reach early adulthood.

Values can be differentiated from attitudes as follows:

Values	*Attitudes*
1. Very deep seated	1. Surface oriented
2. Once developed, rarely change (and if changed, seldom drastically)	2. Are not as long term and will change over time
3. Are few in number	3. Are many in number
4. Are more "global" and represent a system of beliefs about broad issues	4. Are more specific; relate targeted issues and/or people
5. Guide attitudes and behvior	5. Are guided by values
6. Can be negative or positive (in a social/moral/religious sense)	6. Can be negative or positive

Senior managers and executives should routinely engage in value clarification; that is, they should reflect upon what their values are and whether their behaviors (as well as their careers and present positions) are consistent or inconsistent with those values. Conflict between values and behaviors can have many negative outcomes, including the inability to perform a job to the extent needed, the inability to follow appropriate behavior/protocols, and possibly job loss. Perhaps a more disturbing outcome would be cognitive dissonance, a psychological conflict that occurs when beliefs and actions are contradictory.

Cornerstones of an Executive Value System

A strong work ethic is a crucial aspect of an executive value system. Senior managers should enjoy hard work and the sense of pride that comes with accomplishments. Persons who have a strong work ethic and are working at jobs they enjoy (often a requisite component of a strong work ethic) take pleasure in coming to work each day. Their work provides meaning for their lives and enhances their psychological well-being. Related to a strong work ethic is the desire for meaningful involvement, a value that is prevalent among health care executives. People in health care tend to seek ways of contributing to the well-being of others and are committed to working for a greater good.

Another crucial aspect of an executive value system, achievement motivation, is related to a strong work ethic. Executives must be persons who get things done. They must be driven and motivated by seeing positive changes made within their organizations. Persons who are motivated by achieving goals emphasize setting and achieving objectives and then going on to set new goals. They place a heavy emphasis on personal growth.

A third crucial aspect of an executive value system is a genuine respect for other people. Many successful executives have achieved their positions because of their regard and esteem for others, in that they did not manipulate people for their own personal gain but instead helped others develop in ways that ultimately aided their own causes. Such people often have a strong desire to "make a contribution," whether to an organization, to other people, or to society. They make an effort to "give something back." The late Woody Hayes, the colorful and oftentimes controversial former football coach at Ohio State University, frequently said, "You can never pay anyone back for helping you—you can only pay forward."

Servant leadership—the concept that leaders do not control those who follow them but simply serve their followers and meet their needs—is another crucial executive value. Servant leadership is powerful in that because the emphasis is on serving the needs of the followers, those followers grow and develop through the efforts of their leaders and achieve more as a result. They are typically more loyal because they know that the manager is focused on their needs rather than his or her own. In practical, day-to-day terms, executives who practice servant leadership see their role as path clearing for their staff. They focus their energies on making the jobs of their subordinates easier. Servant leadership will be discussed in detail in Chapter 7.

In addition to the "cornerstones" of an executive value system, there are three essential qualities—honesty, credibility, and integrity—that are the most important components of an executive value system and are absolutely critical for executive success. Because of their importance, the protocols discussed in this book will emphasize them heavily.

Honesty

A CFO of a small hospital was convicted of supervising the double-billing of Medicaid accounts. At another hospital, the CEO and CFO padded the financial forecasts when going for a bond rating. A vice president for corporate financial services listed "doctored" numbers on a report that was presented to the corporate board. The board's decisions involved several strategic resolutions based upon the original numbers, which were changed later for the auditors. A vice president of facilities support services had his house painted by a couple of maintenance people and then added additional hours on their time cards in order to pay them. A senior vice president was reimbursed for travel by a state trade association and then turned in the same expenses to his employer for reimbursement. These are only a few examples of dishonest health care executives who exploit their positions for personal gain.

How does this differ from the discussion on ethics? In some ways, it does not. Protocols can suggest appropriate, ethical behavior, but many ethical issues involve problems and questions that do not always have clear-cut answers and solutions. For many questions with ethical dimensions, there are indeed several different approaches to the solutions. The deeper discussion of values, in Chapter 6, will be helpful to readers formulating their own approaches to ethical decision making.

Senior managers and executives must be truthful; their words must be their bond. The wrong words, especially untruths, can permanently damage executives' character and their ability to lead and influence others.

Untruthfulness can take many forms, but should be avoided in all forms. The following are forms of untruthfulness that are, unfortunately, all too common in management.

Distortion

This is frequently used by management today, especially to help sell a position or a proposal. Consider the many presentations that contain warnings about extreme or unlikely implications. Distortion can also apply to that which is left unsaid. Often key details are left out that might sway decisions.

Insinuation

Many managers will introduce ideas in a covert manner, thinking that they can persuade team members individually more successfully than they could convince the whole group of the merits of their idea. This is often done in one-on-one meetings with team members in the hopes of influencing later group deliberations.

Exaggeration

Similar to distortion, this has become almost acceptable within management circles. Consider the number of times that health care executives claim about one issue or another, "This will endanger patient care." Then consider how few times such a claim can be backed up with facts and figures. This is not to say that senior managers should not be concerned with patient care. However, too many times exaggerated claims of patient endangerment are used to further an executive's personal agenda.

It is most unfortunate that untruthfulness has become second nature for many managers. In fact, in many cases, senior-level managers may no longer be aware that they are bending the facts.

On very rare occasions it may be permissible to bend the truth in order to protect another person. For example, telling a person that he or she looks great (or has made a good effort in their work) even if that is not strictly true may be appropriate when the situation calls for boosting him or her up. Or if someone asks how things are going, it may be appropriate to respond positively even though this is not true in order to maintain some positive morale.

A lot of the issues pertaining to truthfulness call for personal judgment on the part of executives. Many senior managers avoid answering questions directly, especially when they do not know the answers or when they want to keep information away from others.

Untruthfulness comes in many forms and is pervasive within the work environment. Successful and effective executives, however, honor truth and attempt to practice it. This will go a long way in developing and maintaining integrity and honesty.

Credibility

Credibility is an important executive value because it is how leaders convince others to follow them. Credibility is determined by the extent to which those working for and with senior managers and executives (superiors, peers, and subordinates) believe that they will do what they say they will.

As managers climb higher in organizations, they actually become *less accountable* to people. This makes it easier for them to lose credibility because their activities are not monitored by others to the same extent as those of others who are lower in hierarchy. Consider the reality of executive life. Although the negative outcomes of not being accountable are certainly greater for senior managers, and the potential costs to their organizations are greater as well, there is less pressure on them on a day-to-day basis. Front-line employees work almost constantly in the presence of their supervisors. Employees are frequently monitored and observed. This is not so with senior managers.

As a result of this independence, senior managers are able to promise more to more people, particularly subordinates, and then are often able to disregard or overlook the necessity of following through on those promises. This undermines their credibility.

Some guiding principles for gaining and keeping credibility are discussed below.

Promise Only What Can Be Done

Executives should be cautious about promising (or even suggesting) that they can or will do certain things. If they say they will do something, then they must do it. They should avoid situations where representations are made but not precisely fulfilled. These include informing subordinates that certain policies will be changed and telling superiors that a certain report will be delivered at a certain time. This goes to the heart of credibility.

Remember That Credibility Is an All-or-None Proposition

There is no such thing as 85 percent credibility or 92 percent credibility—one either has 100 percent credibility or no credibility. If unacceptable behavior reduces a manager's credibility to nothing, the manager will fail.

Say No When Necessary

We all tend to want to please others and tell them what they want to hear. Few people really like saying no. Often senior managers will put people off by saying that they will "get back" to them even though they already know that the answer they will give will not be what the person wants to hear. This raises expectation levels falsely and often causes others to misperceive that a promise or guarantee was made. Remember, as was discussed above, executives who say they will do something *must do it*. If they cannot do it, then they must be very careful to explain why.

Keep a List of Promises

Many successful executives keep a written record of promises they make. A well-known CEO who was known for his thorough follow-through once said, "If you say you will do something, *write it down*. No one person's mind is large enough to store all the promises made during a typical work week."

Follow Up on Everything

Executives should be certain to follow up with people. This should be approached with the same intensity as preparing for a board meeting or a job interview.

Admit Mistakes

Senior managers and executives should admit errors of omission or commission. There is nothing wrong with showing that they are indeed human and make errors in judgment or other mistakes.

A hospital vice president made a $45,000 error in personnel costs when computing a budget. He realized that there was a good chance that the error would be overlooked, so he could get away with not informing the CFO and the CEO, for the budget had already been approved by the board. He knew that sometime during the year the error might surface but felt that with overtime and other variable expenses the size of the error would not seem that great. Also, he believed there was a good chance that the error might not be noticed at all. Nonetheless, the vice president decided to reveal the error to the CFO and the CEO, taking full personal responsibility for it. To his surprise, both reacted quite positively, and the CFO came up with a solution that minimized the potential impact of the error.

Integrity

Joseph L. Badaracco, Jr., and Richard R. Ellsworth write in *Leadership and the Quest for Integrity* that "in essence, integrity is consistency between what a manager believes, how a manager acts, and a manager's aspiration for his or her organization."[1] One of the principal functions of senior managers is to ensure that the organization maintains consistency in working toward its goals. The discussion below presents some guiding principles for maintaining high integrity.

Maintain Confidences

Senior managers have access to a great deal of insider information and must honor confidentiality. Confidentiality is especially important when employees provide information or raise issues and concerns about supervisors but wish to remain anonymous. Senior managers must keep the confidentiality of employees as a sacred trust.

Personalize Decisions

Executives sometimes make global decisions for their organizations without considering the impact upon specific individuals. This may occur when action is taken on layoffs or terminations. Executives should attempt to keep issues and problems personalized. By doing this, they can better understand the true human impact of their decisions. The human costs involved in decisions and actions are often the only ones which ultimately make or break plans and programs.

Avoid Temptation

Executives should avoid situations where they may be tempted to do the wrong thing. They should strive to eliminate or minimize potentially risky or compromising situations. One hospital CEO, for example, will not allow a petty cash fund for executive office use because she believes that it creates too much potential for wrongdoing. Many CEOs and CFOs insist on signing off on even minor expenses incurred by senior management officers. By doing this, they help eliminate the possible temptations of expense reimbursement programs.

Establish an Organizationwide Policy on Integrity

Health care administrators should consider establishing specific policies and guidelines that mandate employee integrity. At a minimum, these should include a conflict of interest statement and a policy regarding the acceptance of gratuities. The conflict-of-interest statement should require all senior managers and departmental managers to sign an annual acknowledgment identifying any potential conflicts of interest.

The Executive Value System in Daily Practice

Consider the following daily dilemmas in a senior manager's life.

- Do you ever fail to get back to someone by the date or time you said you would?
- Have you ever inflated an expense account (by even a small amount)?
- Do you ever say "X" and do "Y"? Or say "A" but mean "B"?

- Regardless of your definition of insincerity, are you ever insincere?

It is a rare executive who can honestly say "no" to all of these questions.

The values and integrity of the organization are driven by the values and integrity of the men and women who lead it. Numerous popular management books have decreed which are the best American companies and which ones do right. Such companies have become very strong and powerful within our culture and are the ones that others try to emulate. A market differentiating factor for an organization might be its strong executive value system.

Senior managers seeking to improve their values should consider the following actions:

1. Closely observe the behavior of executive role models. Choose an individual whom others seem to hold in high esteem and try to define what it is about that person that causes others to hold him or her in high regard.

2. Talk to other executives about deep philosophical issues and values. Be open minded in listening to their viewpoints and suggestions for action.

3. Consider becoming a mentor to others. The constant challenges and questions of those for whom you are a mentor will help you to grow and develop as well.

4. Read literature that is not work-related but instead focuses on service to society and self-discipline. Try to determine those elements that make people successful.

This brief chapter is intended to get readers to develop an inner focus that targets the value system that drives their behavior. In many respects, the principles underlying this chapter form the focus for the beginning of behavior change in most of the areas discussed in the remainder of this book. Honesty, credibility, and integrity are characteristics of most successful and effective senior managers and executives. They have values that help them to be worthy of the respect, dignity, and honor accorded their position in society.

Note

1. J. L. Badaracco, Jr., and R. R. Ellsworth, *Leadership and the Quest for Integrity* (Boston: Harvard Business School, 1989), 9.

5

BUILDING ONE'S
PROFESSIONAL REPUTATION

Most senior managers and executives in health care consider themselves to be professionals. However, there is no universal agreement among other professionals that health care administration is in fact a profession. Indeed, many senior managers and executives in health care grapple with the challenge of working with other clearly delineated (at least by society as a whole) *professionals* (such as physicians) who do not always view them as *professionals*.

A profession is comprised of any group of people who work at jobs that possess a common body of knowledge, that have general standards of quality for the work, and that have certain behavioral standards or ethical guidelines for workers to follow. Given this definition, health care administration is indeed a profession and those working within the field can certainly be considered professionals. This chapter suggests ways in which health care senior managers and executives can enhance and strengthen their professional reputations.

One's professional reputation can be built in two areas: within the organization in which one works and outside, in the community. Many things senior managers do within their own organizations form the foundation of their professional reputations. As they achieve major successes for their organizations, others will hold them in higher esteem.

Interestingly, most senior health care leaders think that only *external* (to the organization) activities contribute to their professional reputation. When asked what enhances their reputations, many executives describe their activities in local or state hospital associations, organizations such as the American College of Healthcare Executives, or local service clubs such as Rotary or Lions. Although these activities are important, an appropriate balance should exist between external and internal (within the organization) efforts in reputation building. Senior managers and executives who spend excessive amounts of time in external activities run the risk of neglecting their real responsibilities and may cause problems in their organizations. This book as a whole suggests actions and behaviors that can help improve an executive's professional reputation within his or her organization.

Enhancing One's External Reputation

Be Active in Associations

Executives should actively participate in their own local and state trade associations. They should attend meetings regularly and join committees. Do not speak negatively about such associations; understand their limitations. They serve many diverse sizes and types of institutions and therefore may not be able to meet all the needs of every individual or group within their constituency.

Senior managers and executives should work within the association's framework to address their concerns. They should correspond with the group's senior staff and give them input on issues and lobbying efforts. They should also volunteer to supply facts and specific examples to aid efforts with legislators and other rule makers. Senior managers should serve as a reference source for the association. They should also volunteer to chair and coordinate educational efforts for the association. Doing this provides an opportunity to deal with various leaders in the field who propose new and creative approaches to problems and issues. This will also provide executives with the opportunity to enhance professional development within their geographic area.

Join the American College of Healthcare Executives

Join and support the American College of Healthcare Executives (ACHE). This is not a commercial for that organization but rather a strong suggestion that the successful executive should be involved in the premier organization that represents the health care management profession and credentials health care executives. Executives should strive to progress through the various levels of the ACHE credentialing program. Senior managers can also enhance their reputations by attending the educational sessions offered by the various trade associations and the ACHE. To maximize these educational opportunities, it is important to attend each with a serious intent to learn and participate.

Teach

Senior managers and executives should consider teaching a class in a local college. This allows them to share their knowledge and practical expertise with students and the community.

Support Continuing Research in the Field

An excellent way for executives to enhance their professional reputation is by letting graduate programs in health administration use their organizations as workshops for research. They can also participate in discussions with faculty members and give them practical, experience-based information.

Support Hospital Administration Residency Programs

Executives should support the growth and development of young administrators by sponsoring residents or administrative fellows. This will not only give young future leaders good growth experiences, but it will also enhance the sponsor's professional reputation. Executives can make these experiences meaningful for the residents and fellows by spending time with them and providing structure for their learning.

Share Successes

Some senior managers and executives write articles about their successful programs. They contribute to the literature within the field. They volunteer to lead sessions at educational meetings to tell of their organization's successes.

Provide Legislative Input

Many successful executives analyze proposed legislation and write Congress and state and local legislative bodies to inform them of the impact of legislation on their institutions. They invite local legislators to their institutions at least annually to ensure that they are familiar with them, the organization, and its needs. They should not use the occasion as simply a chance to complain about how laws and regulations are making it difficult to run the institution. Instead, they should propose alternative legislation or action.

Participate in Community and Service Clubs

Executives should be active in community organizations such as the chamber of commerce or Rotary or Lions Club. They should attend meetings regularly and volunteer to help in activities whenever possible.

Executives should remember that not all of their professional reputation is acquired in the health care setting or in health care activities. Many reputation-enhancing activities are related to other industries and areas of society. Participation in community activities also provides an opportunity to identify community needs and gain community support for the health care organization.

Enhancing One's Internal Reputation

The successful executive must strike a balance between external activities and internal concerns. Executives should not become so active outside the organization that they allow their performance within the organization to suffer.

The manager can greatly enhance his or her professional reputation within the organization by following many of the protocols discussed in this book. In addition, a manager's internal reputation frequently is tied to work ethic and the results achieved within the organization. The guidelines presented below can enhance senior managers' reputations within the organization.

Provide Goal-Oriented Leadership

Executives should clearly define the organization's goals and ensure that others around them understand and agree with them. Strong, goal-oriented leaders expend enormous energy in identifying mission and purpose as well as targets and aims. They look for ways to measure progress. Such leaders stay focused on future trends and issues; they seldom spend time lamenting the past. Once their goals are met, they set new and more difficult ones.

These executives are not satisfied with meeting just one set of standards. They believe in ongoing improvement—that things can always be made better.

Successful leaders do not confuse busyness or activity with accomplishments and results. They recognize that people can be quite busy on a day-to-day basis and yet accomplish relatively little. They work hard to ensure that their daily activities are moving their organizations and themselves forward.

In setting goals, successful executives strive to meet several criteria. First, goals must be time-measurable. In other words, progress must be measurable within a particular period of time. Second, goals must be quantifiable; there must be a method for determining whether they have been met. Third, goals must be relevant to the strategic direction of the organization; they must tie into its mission and success parameters.

Catch the "Can Do" Spirit

Executives should attempt to develop a "can do" attitude. They should determine that no problem is insurmountable, no crisis unsolvable. During the 1970s, the patient care administration program at The Ohio State University Hospitals developed a goal against which all efforts were measured. It was simply labeled "can do." This of course was nothing new or terribly sophisticated. However, its positive impact on the organization during those years was enormous. The program itself was a very strong one because of the high commitment level of the team members. They were able to cut through a cumbersome bureaucracy and maintain high standards of quality for their patient care units. A number of the team members have gone on to higher administrative positions. Their success is in part attributable to how they approach issues and problems.

Executives who want to develop a positive personal approach may benefit from programs that address this need. Many successful personal development programs with good track records emphasize a willing "can do" attitude. This foundation can help executives build a winning attitude in themselves and their organization. One successful COO of a midwestern hospital has a sign on his desk that says "Just do it." He uses this theme to help move on with problem solving and addressing the issues of the day for his organization.

Consider which individuals in organizations are usually given extra projects and responsibilities. They are typically the ones with "can do" attitudes. The organization's pessimists and naysayers are seldom placed in authority roles and rarely participate in helping organizations make major strides forward. The premise in manufacturing that output is a function of input can also be applied to individuals.

Take Credit When Credit Is Due

Executives should take appropriate credit for the good work that they do. If others do not know about a person's accomplishments, they cannot assign him or her appropriate additional career-enhancing duties.

Participate Actively in All Areas of the Organization

Senior administrative staff members should be active in committee meetings. They should attend various meetings, such as medical staff meetings, on a regular basis.

Executives should also be active and visible within the various employee areas of the organization. Many executives develop a positive reputation with the staff and physicians by maintaining high visibility, being available to help, and always being interested in others' concerns. They are always positive and upbeat about their organization, their areas of responsibility, and the things that others are doing for their organizations. They become known as problem solvers and bureaucracy busters.

Senior managers should consider serving as mentors to department heads and staff managers. They may want to spend time with as many managers as possible in arenas other than traditional staff meetings and one-to-one meetings. Doing this increases their personal influence.

Be Punctual

Successful executives complete tasks on time or early. For many executives this is an obsession. The timely completion of assigned or promised work is a major factor in maintaining credibility.

Sell Ideas

Senior managers and executives should develop the art of selling their ideas. Most day-to-day work is done through the process of developing, presenting, and selling ideas and concepts. The ability to influence and persuade is critical in executive success.

Give some thought to this different approach to the presentation of proposals and concepts. Start the proposal with the end statement of desired activity, then provide the details supporting the proposal. This approach is effective because most people wonder what a proposal is going to be if it takes a while to surface during a presentation. They will then make an assumption about what it is and decide whether they are in favor of or against it. If they make the wrong assumption, then they become lost in the presentation. If they make the correct assumption, they may decide against the proposal before hearing all of the facts.

Senior managers can enhance their negotiation skills by being thoroughly prepared with facts and alternative solutions to issues. They should also be prepared to compromise on various issues of concern.

Be an Organizational Cheerleader

Many very successful senior managers are well known within their organizations as cheerleaders. They are always ready to help junior managers find solutions to their problems. They contribute by their teamwork to the good of the entire organization. They keep spirits up and encourage a positive outlook toward problems and concerns.

Enjoying What One Does

To build positive professional reputations, executives must truly enjoy what they do. It is quite evident to those both within and outside the organization that those who relish their work are usually those who have the finest reputations.

The health care field is challenging and requires more than just stamina and knowledge. Its managers must enjoy seeing the results of their efforts. They must also enjoy knowing that their contributions are being felt within and outside their institutions.

Lou Holtz, the head football coach at Notre Dame University, has given many speeches about how personal reputations are made. He focuses on the importance of enjoying working with others, noting that there are three key questions that people should ask in any relationship:

1. Can I trust you?
2. Are you committed to excellence?
3. Do you care about me?

Holtz believes that in order to live by these principles, people must absolutely enjoy what they do. This is not to suggest that a position must always be easy and happy, but in order to enhance effectiveness, senior managers must find some satisfaction in their jobs.

This satisfaction has two foundations. The first is high self-esteem. Those with high self-esteem have confidence in what they do. They are enthusiastic about getting up each morning and going to work and are willing to take on additional tasks for the organization. Such people smile and encourage others around them.

The second foundation is contentment with one's profession. Contented professionals are glad that they have chosen their careers. They spend time talking to others about the joy and excitement their career brings them. If one does not feel this way, one should find a more satisfying profession. As one senior finance officer of a health care organization put it, "For those who think that this field (health care) is too tough and frustrating, please get out—I do not want them to ruin it for the rest of us with their negative attitudes and behavior."

Summary

Building a professional reputation is not merely creating a facade. A very successful vice president of operations at a teaching hospital was asked how he had developed such a strong reputation. He replied, "I was just doing my job." The things that he did were needed in order to help the organization progress and provided support to those around him.

6

ETHICS FOR HEALTH CARE EXECUTIVES

Ethics in business is at long last being studied in the leading graduate schools of business across the country and is now a frequent topic in business journals and magazines. A number of authors have contributed to the heightened interest in the subject. Kenneth Blanchard and Norman Vincent Peale's *The Power of Ethical Management* is an excellent book and has been widely read.[1] Many business seminars today even provide some mention, albeit brief, of ethical issues.

In health care circles, however, discussions of ethics seem relegated to such medical-legal ethical issues as abortion, euthanasia, living wills, the rationing of health care, and parenteral nutrition. Although health care practitioners should continue to consider these important issues, they should not be the only focus of ethics in health care.

Health care is probably more value-driven than any other industry. The obligations to patients within the healing and caring environment are examples of the highest calling within society. A strong emphasis on managerial ethics is an appropriate corollary to this societal obligation and responsibility.

Health care institutions tend to follow one another's lead. When one hospital innovates a service or program, others soon add it. If one hospital acquires a certain piece of equipment, not long afterward a nearby hospital will purchase the same equipment. When one hospital in an area begins to advertise, most of the others follow. In human resources, when one organization adds a benefit or a special wage differential, the others in the area do the same. If one begins to develop a special product line, such as women's services, the others get on the bandwagon.

The result is that health care organizations tend to seem alike to the public. When this happens in any industry (not just health care) successful organizations do something to differentiate themselves. For example, a health care organization might differentiate itself by emphasizing its strong managerial ethics. A health care organization with a strong ethical orientation might be able to send a different message to its consumers, physicians, and employees. As a result of this differentiation, the organization may become more successful than its competitors. This market differentiation of ethical leadership must start at the senior management level. Obviously, the increase of market share should not be the reason for the development of an ethical environment. Health care organizations should be ethical if for no other reason than that it is right.

Executives who want to make their organizations stand out from the others must constantly try to set appropriate examples. They must be willing to conduct themselves as if someone were watching all the time. The belief that one can get away with unethical behavior because no one is watching or because some act really will not hurt anyone can damage careers.

This chapter sets forth several guiding principles that can help senior managers make more ethical decisions.

Ethics within the context of this discussion simply means the standards that help people make right decisions rather than wrong ones. There is no effort to address issues involving religion or morality. The protocols presented in this chapter are intended to help senior managers and executives make appropriate ethical choices and decisions.

Blanchard and Peale suggest a slightly elementary approach to ethical issues in this statement: "There is no right way to do a wrong thing."[2] Unfortunately, ethical issues are often much more complex than this, and it is well known that managers often disagree on which course of action to take.

Approaching Ethics from Three Angles

Senior managers need to approach ethical issues from three angles. First, they should follow the ethical guidelines or policies promulgated by the organization in which they work. Second, they should adhere to any ethical code of conduct or standards set forth by a professional organization. Third, and most important, they should maintain those standards that ethical individuals use for decision making.

Organizational Codes of Ethics

Many organizations, through their codes of conduct, prescribe an organizational code of ethics that is either developed by a committee of the board of trustees or authored by the CEO. The mission statement of an organization may also include references to ethical behavior. It may also include a policy statement that refers to the desirability of ethical conduct.

Too often, however, these written statements are ignored because they do not set forth any specific behavioral expectations.

Those in positions of power and influence (primarily the trustees and the CEO) should establish and publish clearly written ethical standards for their organizations. At a minimum, an organization should have a published policy on the acceptance of gifts and gratuities.

Corporately prescribed ethical behavior does not stop with individual behavior; it should include guidelines for organizational responses. There are a number of excellent examples of corporate ethical conduct. Perhaps the best is the way in which McNeil, the maker of Tylenol, responded to the poisoned capsules that killed several people. McNeil immediately recalled all products from the shelves, offered money-back guarantees on returned products, set up a toll-free response number, and quickly pioneered new packaging techniques. This was done at great expense but was viewed as a highly ethical response. Health care organizations should be prepared to respond quickly and ethically in the event of a crisis.

Professional Codes of Ethics

Professionals should follow the guidelines of their professional codes of ethics. One of the marks of a profession is the existence of such a code. These codes, however, are only as good as the sanctions set up to enforce them and the willingness of the members of the profession to sincerely subscribe to them and police themselves.

Readers should become familiar with the ethical code of the American College of Healthcare Executives. This should be done for reasons other than passing the ACHE membership exam! This code prescribes general principles that should be of great use to the health care executive. The ethical tenets that are set forth form a worthy set of guiding principles for health care executives. They address many of the more global ethical dilemmas faced by executives and suggest appropriate behavior.

Conflict of interest is one of the most difficult ethical areas. The ACHE code of ethics has an excellent discussion on this topic. It advises executives to conduct themselves in the best interests of the organizations they serve, to accept no gifts offered to sway decisions, and to advise authorities of internal and external conflict of interest situations.

Ethical Decision-Making Standards

In their book *Leadership and the Quest for Integrity*, Joseph J. Badaracco, Jr., and Richard R. Ellsworth sum up the issue of personal involvement in ethical decision making as follows:

Leadership in a world of dilemmas is not, fundamentally, a matter of style, charisma, or professional management technique. It is a difficult daily quest for integrity. Managers' behavior should be an unadorned, consistent reflection of what they believe and what they aspire to for a company. Managers who take this approach earn trust. Commitment to leadership through integrity can help managers through the inevitable periods of anxiety, doubt, and trial, and give them a sense of priorities to guide them through an uncertain world.[3]

Badaracco and Ellsworth suggest that the situational approach to management (that is, that every decision depends upon the demands of the situation) is not always appropriate for truly effective leadership. There are certain ethical situations which demand consistent responses over time.

In the final analysis, ethical managers are the most effective and contribute the most. Because their personal interests are consistent with the needs of their organization, their behavior will not result in a fatal flaw that harms their leadership effectiveness. Being ethical does not mean that someone is always right. Nor does it mean that in every situation the decision one makes or the action one takes is inviolate. What it means in this context is that:

1. Senior managers should give serious consideration to the ethical implications of their decisions.

2. Senior managers should have a personal code of ethics that they will not violate in decision making.

3. Decisions should be made relative to the good they provide to groups of people as a whole and not only for the benefit of the individual.

The protocols for ethical behavior discussed below attempt to establish *absolutes*. In a world dealing with ethical imperatives, there is no such thing as "grading on the curve." Ethical behavior falls into an "either-or" category, it either is or is not ethical. Although in managerial life answers are not always easy and clear-cut, it is necessary to set forth principles that allow no leeway or license. These principles are intended to assist in increasing ethical behavior.

Some readers may take exception to the protocols discussed below because they do not wish to see certain absolutes set forth. This chapter more than any other in the book sets forth conclusive and definitive actions for situations. It is hoped that readers will use it to try to improve their conduct when making decisions in which the *right* approach is not clear.

Ethical Protocols in the Office

Use of Office Stationery and Postage

Senior managers should not use office stationery and postage for personal correspondence. This is particularly true if they are involved in a job search. Cover letters and résumés should not be sent on company letterhead and using the company postage meter. Different rules may apply in outplacement situations, however.

Use of Petty Cash

If there is an office petty cash fund, its use must be clearly documented, and senior managers must avoid any personal use of these funds. It is best not to provide anyone access to this type of petty cash fund without some approval mechanism.

Use of Copy Machines

A mechanism should be set up to allow senior managers to pay for their personal copying, unless of course this is specifically spelled out as an executive benefit.

Personal Long-Distance Telephone Calls

Ethical senior managers should keep track of their personal long-distance telephone calls and reimburse the organization for them.

Use of Secretaries for Personal Errands

Unless senior managers own the company, their secretaries work for the company and not for them personally. This means that asking them to do personal errands and perform other personal services is not appropriate. The spouses of senior managers and executives also should not expect secretaries to do personal tasks or run errands for them.

This applies to all subordinates of senior managers. Staff members should not be expected to do personal chores for senior executives. For example, a member of the maintenance staff should not be asked to perform maintenance tasks at an executive's home during work hours.

An example of unethical and inappropriate use of staff occurred at a midwestern hospital where several trees were cut down on hospital property.

The groundskeepers were instructed to cut the wood into fireplace-sized logs and deliver half to the CEO's home and half to the COO's home.

General Ethical Protocols

Keep Information Confidential

Comments made in confidence must be kept confidential. People who give information have the right to expect you to observe their wishes for confidentiality. However, sometimes observing strict confidentiality prevents an executive from taking action to solve a problem.

One approach to this dilemma is to remind the individual requesting confidentiality that if the statements must be kept in strict confidence, nothing can really be done about solving the problem or ameliorating the situation. Executives should be certain they do not leave the impression that they can or will do something in these cases. This will temper the expectations of the person sharing the information as well as protect the confidentiality of that informant.

Do Not Accept Anything of Value

Executives should avoid accepting *anything* from people with whom they have business relationships.

This protocol is probably the one most frequently violated by senior managers; most people make exceptions to this rule. The exceptions usually involve allowing consultants or others to buy lunches or dinners or accepting small gifts from vendors or others. The potential problem with this is knowing where to draw the line. This problem can be avoided by never accepting anything—including a free lunch—from business associates. However, most executives find this a difficult, if not impossible, precedent to set. In some instances, it may even threaten a good business relationship.

Do Not Misuse Company Property

The organization's equipment and supplies are for business use, not personal use. Books, tape recorders, and other items bought with the organization's funds for use in one's work should only be used for that purpose.

Do Not Take Credit for Other's Work

When subordinates do work that is well received, it is only correct for managers to give credit where credit is due. Subordinates should also know that they have received credit.

Practice What You Preach

Executives should follow their own rules as well as those of their organizations. Although much of this is common sense, there is an ethical dimension to it as well. For example, executives should not expect to have their paychecks released early when other employees do not have the same opportunity, and executives should be careful to park in the correct spaces. One hospital had a temporary parking shortage and asked all employees to park on surface lots several blocks from the hospital. Although the hospital president had a reserved space in the parking garage, during the shortage he parked in the less convenient off-site lots along with the rest of the employees.

In many organizations, unethical practices result from a sense of executive privilege ("rank has its privileges"). A middle manager worked in an organization where all middle managers were to work as if they were paid on an hourly basis, although their hours were not monitored as such. This particular middle manager took time off every two weeks to get a haircut, which he justified to himself by explaining, "It grows on hospital time! I'll get it cut on hospital time." Although this example is extreme—few hospitals have their managers working on an hourly basis—the meaning is pertinent.

Act as if Someone Is Always Watching

Executives should consider themselves to be always under scrutiny and be able to justify their actions in ethical terms. An executive's reputation and credibility are *always* subject to challenge. He or she should never let the guard down. Most readers would agree that nothing is worse than being called unethical.

When in Doubt, Do Not Do It

If there is ever any doubt about whether an action is ethical, senior managers and executives should refrain from that action, if possible. When in doubt, do not do it.

Summary

The entire area of ethics raises many questions and answers few. Perhaps this is good. It is often through raising questions that correct answers are sought and developed. However, at times this leaves health care managers without a general sense of direction. The following general protocol guidelines can be used in approaching ethical dilemmas:

- The ultimate enemy, the one that causes most unethical behavior, is selfishness. Senior managers who wish to lead ethical lives should strive to be less selfish. Giving to others and being willing to share will ward off a lot of behavior which borders on the unethical.

- Senior managers and executives should attempt to have as one of their life goals making a contribution to society when making decisions, their guiding ethical principle should be to take actions that cause the greatest good for the greatest number of people (although certainly there are exceptions to this rule). Service provided within the health care environment is service that should be viewed by society as being on a higher order than that of other areas of business and industry.

- Perhaps the best ethical guidelines are the ones developed by Rotary International: think, say, and do what is truthful, fair, builds good will, and is beneficial to all concerned. Executives should be selfless, contribute to society, give to others, uphold truth and fairness, and seek better relationships. All these actions will add up to a more ethical executive lifestyle.

Notes

1. K. Blanchard and N. V. Peale, *The Power of Ethical Management* (New York: William Morrow, 1988).
2. Ibid., 19.
3. J. L. Badaracco, Jr., and R. R. Ellsworth, *Leadership and the Quest for Integrity* (Boston: Harvard Business School Press, 1989), 209.

Further Readings

American College of Healthcare Executives. *Code of Ethics*. Chicago: American College of Healthcare Executives, 1992.
Griffith, J. R. *The Moral Challenges of Health Care Management*. Ann Arbor, MI: Health Administration Press, 1993.

PART II

SERVING OTHERS

7

INTERPERSONAL RELATIONSHIPS

Successful executive managers should be able to get along with others and influence, persuade, and inspire them. These interpersonal skills are seldom taught, rarely discussed, and infrequently included in management development programs or senior management development programs. They are seldom addressed in business journals or periodicals.

In the past several years increasing emphasis has been placed on the need to improve interpersonal skills. Much of this emphasis began in management with the advent of Tom Peters's "excellence" revolution. Management speakers and trainers talked about the power that rested within people and the need to get along with others as well as traditional approaches to team building. The *Wall Street Journal* described the efforts of the accounting firm Arthur Andersen to improve interpersonal skills in an article on December 14, 1990: "Arthur Andersen is one of many companies placing new emphasis on 'people skills' for their managers and executives. In the past, even ordinary managers could succeed by just knowing the business. But increasingly, managers with 'people conflicts' are being sent to school to learn how to relate better to others."

Interpersonal skills are difficult to teach because they are not easily quantifiable. Management tends to avoid focusing on that which is not concrete and objective. In most organizations, as long as the measurable portions were going well, success is thought to be evident and all other factors are ignored. Even union organizational efforts are seldom viewed as problems resulting from interpersonal skills issues.

The excellence movement led by Tom Peters, with its corresponding emphasis on interpersonal skills and conflict management, began with his book *In Search of Excellence*. One of his keys to excellence in organizations was in how people were treated. "Treat people as adults. Treat them as partners; treat them with dignity; treat them with respect. Treat them—not capital spending and automation—as the primary source of productivity gains."[1]

Most senior managers or executives would agree that the ability to get along with people is one of the successful executive's most important skills. However, they seem to have trouble putting that belief into action. The following observations are based on hundreds of formal and informal interviews, reviews of more than 15 organizational attitude surveys, and professional consultation with more than 5,200 managers:

- Many employees fear their senior leadership. They feel intimidated by them and seldom see them as real people.

- Employees who talk honestly about their feelings toward top management speak with disgust and aversion.

- Many attitude surveys today show that senior management in all companies has less credibility than ever before.

- Most senior managers are so distant from the employee population that they have little sense of what is really occurring in the organization.

- Many senior managers actually feel uncomfortable with employees.

These problem areas focus on relationships with subordinates. However, good interpersonal skills are also important in dealing with peers and superiors. Here the ability to get along is often as important for the senior manager's job as getting results.

There are no proven methods for developing stronger interpersonal skills. The protocols discussed below, however, can help improve interpersonal relationships.

Show Sincere Respect for Human Dignity

Having true and sincere respect for human dignity makes the acquisition and maintenance of good interpersonal skills somewhat effortless. Senior managers and executives who truly honor and hold in high esteem *all* people (not just those who are like themselves or who serve them well) will find that interpersonal skills come naturally.

Acquiring good interpersonal skills depends upon selflessness and a willingness to often (if not always) put others ahead of oneself.

Good interpersonal skills are predicated on

- a warm and sympathetic attitude toward others;
- a willingness to give and share;

- a willingness (*and* ability) to see good in all others; and
- a desire to make others feel comfortable.

These result from having respect and regard for other people and from treating others as one treats oneself. However, it is frequently difficult for executives to give of themselves because of the intense competitive spirit that brought them to their present positions.

Protocols for Improving Interpersonal Skills

All of these protocols are based upon compassion for and sensitivity to others. Stephen Strasser, in *Working It Out: Sanity and Success in the Workplace*, states that, "The soul of effective interpersonal relations is empathy. Empathetic managers and employees express to others a sense of understanding and compassion for their emotions and feelings."[2]

As senior managers and executives interact with others, they should consider and try to understand others' attitudes, feelings, dreams, and fears. Their goal should be to influence others to help in organizational endeavors. Senior managers can build closer and more productive relationships by showing empathy, understanding, and acceptance. They should have a warm and sympathetic attitude toward others. The protocols discussed below relate to this.

Avoid Favoritism

Executives should work hard to avoid showing favoritism. Favoritism breeds dissension, resentment, and unhealthy competition. Senior managers especially cannot afford to be perceived by others as having favorites. If they are, a popular topic on the organizational grapevine will be the identification of who is "in" and who is "out" with senior-level bosses, which will distract the organization from making positive strides toward its goals.

Be Direct

Executives should try to be honest and aboveboard with others. They should strive to be known as persons who are direct, forthright, and candid. Such people are known on the company grapevines as "straight shooters." This unfailing candor and straightforwardness helps develop and maintain good interpersonal relationships.

Maintain One-to-One Relationships

When possible, senior managers should deal with people face to face; good interpersonal relationships are person-to-person. The intimacy and rapport that evolve from a one-to-one personal encounter help to nullify negative feelings. With rare exceptions, negative feelings can be minimized or at least redirected toward a positive outcome. When dealing with people face to face one can read their body language and facial expressions, which enhances communication and understanding. Busy executives should resist the temptation in today's fast-paced environment to telephone instead of visiting people. They should take the time to walk to the offices and work locations of others. During face-to-face encounters, executives should maintain eye contact. These simple but important actions will help build stronger interpersonal relationships.

Be Consistent

Executives should not be two-faced. They should say and mean the same things to everyone. Executives should behave as if everything they say and do is videotaped and then played back for all to see. They should follow through on promises and strive to be as consistent as possible.

Use Criticism Carefully and Constructively

If it is necessary to offer criticism managers should do so in private. This is very simple and basic, and yet it is often violated by senior managers and executives, especially in staff meetings. Some managers feel that if their criticism is not formal discipline, then it can be done in front of other peer-level persons. Sometimes such comments may not be intended as actual criticism but instead as targeted, motivational barbs. Some executives may also believe that group discussion with negative comments made in an open meetings is a managerial rite of passage. They may feel that if their managers cannot understand and take the comments, then they should not be in managerial positions. Senior managers would do well to remember the effect these barbs had on them as they climbed the corporate ladder. It is a rare executive who would admit to appreciating and benefiting from this type of criticism.

One midwestern CEO who had just arrived at his new position used scathing criticism to some of the existing senior managers. In doing so, he lost two of the stronger members of his team. Although this was his intention, in the process he alienated other managers whom he wanted to keep, and eventually they left as well.

Another CEO brought four of his vice presidents into his office following their presentations at a board meeting and screamed at them for what he considered to be poor presentations. Three of these executives were gone within a year.

People should be told *why* they are being criticized. Executives should be specific and outline specific *behavior* rather than general personal characteristics. When criticizing, they should offer assistance to the person being criticized and should be certain that the criticism is constructive. Employees should know that their managers want them to succeed. Executives should not follow up their criticism of poor job performances by stepping in and doing the work themselves.

Protocols for Improving Interpersonal Relationships with Subordinate Managers

An executive's immediate subordinates, who usually are managers themselves, are important contributors to his or her success. Those who work directly for senior managers serve as "extensions" or surrogates for them and to a great extent reflect the drive and goal orientation of their superior. An executive's team becomes increasingly important as he or she climbs the organizational ladder because the higher in rank the executive is, the more power and influence his or her subordinates have.

Unfortunately, though, senior managers do not always show their subordinate managers the same respect and consideration that they show to lower-level subordinates. This may be because the work of the more senior manager itself is of greater variety and subordinate managers typically are experts within their own fields. For example, managers of finance, nursing, or human resources are experts in their fields to the CEO. To the vice president of operations, the managers of respiratory therapy, radiology, or dietetics are experts. This difference in perspective can cause misunderstandings about issues that can harm interpersonal relationships. The impact on the subordinate manager may be greater, but the stakes involved are higher for senior managers. Thus, it is crucial that senior managers cultivate good interpersonal relationships with their subordinate managers. The following true stories show why these are critical to managerial success.

- The CEO of a southern hospital would frequently lose his temper in such an explosive fashion that his vice presidents spent vast amounts of time covering for one another's mistakes and hiding negative news so as to avoid his outbursts. When they were included in the interview process for recruitment efforts for peer-level colleagues, they would describe in detail for the candidates the explosive nature of this CEO. As a result, several good candidates who might otherwise have joined the hospital staff rejected offers of employment.

- The CFO of a midwestern teaching hospital had a tendency to stare intently at people who were talking to him. His staring made most people feel very uncomfortable, especially since he did not speak or respond in any other way to the person who was addressing him. After a person finished talking, the CFO let several seconds of silence elapse before responding. Some of his subordinates often wondered whether or not he was listening. Others simply felt that his staring and silence were forms of psychological intimidation. Because his subordinates were uncomfortable with him, the CFO received very little supplemental information from them. Without complete information the value of his decision making was decreased.

- When a vice president of nursing at an eastern hospital was making her rounds, she would frequently call nurse managers together and berate them for rather small issues, such as carts or equipment being left in the halls of the unit. At all other times and places, this vice president seemed to be a good listener and a fair manager. These dressing-down sessions occurred only when she toured the nursing units. Seeing their managers openly criticized had a negative impact on the rest of the unit staff.

- The CEO at a large teaching hospital would frequently ask his subordinates about their families and personal lives. However, after they responded, he would quickly change the subject back to work-oriented issues. It was quite apparent to his subordinates that his interest was not genuine. He was perceived as someone who showed a personal interest in employees only when he needed something from them.

Subordinates are among the most important resources senior managers have. They should be treated accordingly and shown the utmost respect. It is part of the burden of leadership that the responsibility for developing and maintaining good interpersonal relationships rests more with senior managers than subordinates. Subordinates' desire and ability to perform is strongly influenced by how their senior managers relate to them. The protocols described below will help build strong interpersonal relationships with subordinate managers.

Show Concern for Subordinate Managers' Personal and Professional Well-Being

Senior executives and managers should take a sincere interest in their subordinate managers' needs and goals, both personal and professional. Many of the most successful senior leaders in health care have nurtured the careers of subordinates who have gone on to become heads of other organizations. These leaders know that helping subordinates to grow and advance builds a strong network of support and encourages loyalty and diligence from those individuals who are working for them.

Do Not Humiliate Managers

Executives should be careful not to mock or humiliate subordinates either privately or in front of others. Such behavior is extremely destructive to interpersonal relationships.

Take a Personal Interest in Subordinates

Senior managers should get to know their subordinate managers and learn about their families, their problems, and their interests. Showing this level of concern encourages loyalty and forms a foundation for good interpersonal relationships. Although it is important to maintain a comfortable professional distance from employees, it is likewise essential to show them that they are valued as individuals.

Show Tact and Diplomacy

Senior managers must always treat their subordinates with tact and diplomacy. They must show consideration for and sensitivity to their feelings and concerns.

Support Subordinate Managers

Senior managers should provide subordinates with the support and information they need to do their jobs. They should not withhold information as a technique for keeping power.

Managers should not appear to use subordinates for personal gain. They should seriously consider their ideas and help them understand why if their proposals are rejected.

Solicit "Performance Reviews" from Subordinates

Senior executives and managers can get meaningful feedback on their leadership abilities by asking subordinates to review their performances. Questionnaires and formal interviews can be especially helpful in getting useful feedback on leadership style, strengths, and weaknesses. A good time to obtain such feedback is just before a senior manager leaves an organization for another position. Robert Shaver, a leading health care administrator, believes that people are often more willing to appraise and criticize senior managers who are leaving and will reveal things that can help executives evaluate blind spots.

Servant Leadership

In *Servant Leadership*, Robert K. Greenleaf described the concept as follows:

> A fresh critical look is being taken at the issues of power and authority, and people are beginning to learn, however haltingly, to relate to one another in less coercive and more creatively supporting ways. A new moral principle is emerging which holds that the only authority deserving one's allegiance is that which is freely and knowingly granted by the led to the leader in response to, and in proportion to, the clearly evident servant stature of the leader. Those who choose to follow this principle will not casually accept the authority of existing institutions. Rather, they will freely respond only to individuals who are chosen as leaders because they are proven and trusted as servants.[3]

Greenleaf suggests that servant leaders are goal-oriented, tend to listen intently to descriptions of problems to gain a better understanding of them, and are accepting and empathetic in dealing with their subordinates. The essence of servant leadership is a strong drive to develop and maintain positive interpersonal relationships.

Servant leaders do not attempt to manipulate or control subordinates. They encourage an open, honest atmosphere that encourages positive interpersonal relationships.

To practice the principles of servant leadership, senior managers and executives must first look at what their subordinates need in order to do their work. They must share information and assist others to accomplish their goals.

Senior managers who adopt this philosophical approach to subordinates will find that staff members become more supportive in the quest of the goals of the team. They will discover that team members thrive in this kind of environment, relationships will be more positive, and there will be less conflict.

Protocols for Termination

Consider the word *firing*. Given the intrinsic volatility of the word, the act should be handled with great care and reverence. Termination today can be likened to economic capital punishment; it cannot be taken as lightly as perhaps it once was. On a strictly practical level, there are court challenges to and legal tests of the ability to terminate that make it imperative for managers to follow proper procedures.

There are right and wrong ways to discharge employees. The ability to fire is one aspect of an executive's power and authority that should be exercised with great care and sensitivity. Michael Covert, a leading health care executive, once said about firing others, "if it has to be done, do it, but do it with style and treat the person(s) right."

The Appropriate Approach

Terminations are perhaps the toughest test of a manager's interpersonal skills. Even the smallest mistake in handling this volatile situation can have profound ramifications for the employee, the organization, and the executive. The following protocols can aid in approaching termination issues effectively and sensitively.

Do the necessary preparation. Be certain that the decision to terminate is truly necessary and final, but be prepared to respond to information presented by the employee that might alter your decision or the ensuing process. Assemble as many facts and as much evidence as possible. Consider the potential for legal or other challenges.

Follow the proper procedures. The method of termination should be pre-established and consistent across the organization, even for senior-level persons.

Be prepared for any reaction. Managers should give serious consideration to the employee's reaction to being dismissed. Try to anticipate needs, wants, or demands. Little things are important here, including having a supply of tissues available.

Senior managers and executives should not have someone from human resources deliver the final blow. It is the job of the direct supervisor to handle the conversation. There is generally no problem with having another supervisor or a human resources person accompany the manager when handling the conference, but the person who delivers the message should be the one who made the decision.

Consider the timing of terminations. Consider carefully when the actual termination conversation should take place. Both the time of day and the day itself are important. Although there is probably no set rule of thumb to follow, these aspects should be considered:

- Will the person want or need to go back to the work area? Should he or she be accompanied and should the materials removed from the work area be listed and approved?
- Will others be there? Should they see the person right after the termination conversation?

Before allowing the person a number of days or even weeks to close out business activities, executives should carefully consider whether he or she might damage organizational morale or whether sabotage is a possibility.

Most outplacement consultants maintain that the worst time to terminate a person is on Friday. There are several reasons for this. Because the next day is Saturday, it is unlikely that the person will be able to communicate with any business contacts. These contacts are important in that they give the person an immediate outlet, other than family, with whom to discuss the situation and can help terminated employees feel as though they are making some progress toward finding a new position. Friday is also bad in that it gives the person the weekend to brood and become more upset.

Be certain that you are certain. Executives should be prepared for the fact that the employee may provide new information during the course of the termination. They should also be prepared to put the decision to terminate on hold if the new information seems to be pertinent to the decision and may change it. If necessary, executives should tell the employee that the new facts need to be reviewed and a new meeting will be scheduled soon. Be certain then that soon is *soon*; do not become preoccupied with other business and fail to follow through. Avoid having employees sit at home waiting as the senior manager considers new information, investigates new facts, or ponders the decision further.

Be on time. Do not make the employee wait. This is not the time to have a previous meeting run long or to squeeze in a few more return phone calls before holding the termination conversation. In fact, it is often wise to allow some private time to prepare for the termination conference.

Get to the point quickly. A termination meeting is not the time for friendly conversation. Get to the point quickly. The focus of the meeting should be on the termination and only on that. All other conversation is extraneous, including small talk about families, the weather, or sports. This is not to say that the "bullet" should be fired as soon as the person walks into the room. However, the conversation must focus on the issue at hand.

If the termination is unexpected, executives should be prepared for argument, debate, denial, and requests for another chance. They should be humane and allow some of this conversation to occur. However, they should maintain control of the meeting.

Specific Protocols for Dismissing Managers

The protocols discussed below relate specifically to the termination of senior-level management employees. Although these same principles should apply to the termination of employees at all levels, terminations of senior managers tend to attract a lot of attention and require careful planning and preparation. Only rarely is a situation so urgent that is calls for immediate termination without discussion.

Give appropriate warnings. A manager who is dismissed should not be taken by surprise. He or she should have been involved in frank discussions that clearly delineated shortcomings and expectations.

Touch base with appropriate constituencies. Senior managers should determine who, for practical or political reasons, needs to know about the termination in advance. Some board member or key physicians may consider it an affront if they are not notified in advance of certain terminations. However, managers should never forget that confidentiality is paramount in terminations.

Cover any legal considerations. Senior managers should be certain to consider the legal ramifications of the termination. They should review any letters of offer and employment contracts to see that all of their provisions are met. They should not be caught during the termination without all of the pertinent facts. Some executives routinely discuss any terminations with outside legal counsel before acting.

Senior managers should have all of the legally required benefit information available in writing for the terminated employee and present it during the termination conference. If there are benefit options for the terminated employee to exercise, managers should spell those out in writing as well.

Anticipate any questions about salary continuance and benefits and other conditions of employment that may arise. Have answers for all of these questions unless there are choices that the employee must make. In this case, clearly spell out the alternatives.

Many attorneys have standard agreement forms available that cover most termination contingencies. If such forms are used, the person being terminated should be given a form that indicates all of the conditions of the termination. Often the termination/severance agreement includes provisions whereby the employee waives the right to sue. If this is the case, be certain that the agreement is reviewed beforehand by a competent labor attorney.

Prepare for the public announcement of the termination. When managers are dismissed, there should be some discussion with them about the announcement of the dismissal. It may be necessary and appropriate to prepare a news release in some cases. However, the individual's secretary and direct staff must be notified in a more personal manner than the rest of the organization.

Discuss the transition. As much as possible, the senior manager and the dismissed manager should discuss how a smooth transition can be accomplished. They should make plans for handling unfinished projects and ensuring an orderly shift of responsibilities.

Handle the final little details. Senior managers should consider the following small items:

- Return of company keys, ID badges, credit cards, and the like
- Detailing what is contained in certain files
- Arranging for some continuing contact to cover outstanding questions and issues
- Agreement on specific transfer of responsibilities
- Identification of issues and concerns that must be quickly addressed
- Return or purchase of the company car

Be considerate of the terminated manager's secretary. Special consideration should be given to a terminated manager's secretary. Secretaries often have strong allegiances to their supervisors and may be especially upset about the termination and have some difficulty making the transition to a new supervisor.

Consider using outplacement. There has been a great growth in the use of outplacement services in the past several years. If the organization opts to use outplacement, executives should take care to choose a reputable firm (they should not rely solely on the human resources department) and get to know the firm and the counselors who will work with the dismissed employee.

In selecting an outplacement firm, consider the following:

- Do not use firms that expect the terminated employee to pay all or part of the fee. Reputable outplacement firms work only with clients whose former employer pays the entire fee.
- Look for a firm that provides full assessment services and not simply office and telephone backup. Be certain that someone in the organization has visited with the outplacement firm to verify what services it provides.
- Look for a good track record of placing clients in new positions.
- Consider the facilities. The outplacement firm's offices should offer privacy and dignified surroundings to the dismissed employee.
- Make sure that the firm provides ongoing counseling and support.
- Make sure that basic tools and amenities such as out-of-town newspapers, fax machines, copy machines, industry guides, and professional journals and circulars are available.
- Make sure that the firm's counselors show caring and concern for dismissed employees.

The use of a good outplacement firm can often ensure that a termination works out smoothly over the long term. However, it does not excuse executives from their obligation to handle terminations ethically and fairly, and in a manner that maintains the dignity and self-respect of the dismissed employee.

Summary

Good interpersonal skills are indispensable to managers as they climb the organizational ladder and gain authority and responsibility. Unfortunately, however, as executives climb in the organization, they tend to lose sight of the importance of good interpersonal skills. One CEO said that there is a tendency when one achieves high stature within an organization to begin to believe in one's own press clippings. It is at this point that a lot of senior managers forget how they got to the top and neglect the need to continue good interpersonal skills. One executive search firm consultant said that he knew a number of very successful CEOs who had been fired because they lost their skill at getting along with others. Getting along with others is not only necessary; it is a reasonable ethical and moral demand.

To get along with others, it is necessary to practice a certain amount of selflessness; self-centeredness is not conducive to good interpersonal relationships. Giving and sharing are especially important for those in senior-level positions. Executives should contemplate the concept of servant leadership, begin to apply it, and experience how it can provide positive returns in the form of better working relationships.

Notes

1. T. Peters, *In Search of Excellence* (New York: Harper & Row, 1982), 238.
2. S. Strasser, *Working It Out: Sanity and Success in the Workplace* (Englewood Cliffs, NJ: Prentice-Hall, 1988), 173.
3. R. K. Greenleaf, *Servant Leadership* (Mahwah, NJ: Paulist Press, 1977), 9–10.

8

Protocols for Working
with Employees

It is no secret that employees are crucial to the success of any organization. Management literature abounds with references to the importance of having all employees support the mission of the organization. A dedicated, high-quality work force can give an organization an important edge, particularly in health care. Most senior managers and executives would agree that their professional success hinges on their ability to influence their organization's nonprofessional work force. With the growing shortages of registered nurses, allied health technologists, and other key staffers, it is increasingly important to recruit, maintain, and motivate supportive employees.

Not all senior managers and executives are comfortable with their approaches to employees. Some managers are awkward, whereas others tend to act too polished. Because of differences in lifestyle, education, and socioeconomic background, senior managers and executives may feel that they do not have a lot in common with many of their employees. For example, an opportunity to play golf at the executive vice president's private country club could be a very special and prized occasion for employees who play on public golf courses. Senior managers, on the other hand, rarely covet an opportunity to bowl at the local bowling alley. Many executives and managers wear business clothes that are unsuitable for employees' work and are priced beyond their means. There are often differences in where senior managers and employees live, play, socialize, and worship. These differences often separate them and make interpersonal relationships difficult.

Differences in educational and socioeconomic status abound in the work force of the typical health care institution. Often senior managers see employees' family members only at the annual picnic. This is not to suggest that one group in society is "better" than another; however, the reality is that differences between groups of people can make it difficult for them to interrelate.

Even though a senior manager may have come up through the ranks and may feel that his or her roots and feelings are more like those of the employees than those of other senior managers, the differences between executives and the employee population are real. Once an employee is promoted to management, it is hard to continue former relationships and it can be difficult to maintain a close network with former colleagues.

Employees often perceive that managers are insincere or manipulative. This may or may not be true, but remember that the reality for employees, as for most people, is what they perceive. Although many managers will say that they are not insincere or manipulative, that is in fact how they deal with employees. This is often because senior managers have such limited time for meaningful interaction with employees.

In many organizations, the employees may actually *want* to maintain a certain distance from senior management. At one midwestern hospital, several vice presidents tried to work themselves into the employee golf league. They were registered on the substitute list but were never called to play. One of the vice presidents asked an employee in the league why they were never called and was told: "Most of the guys are just not comfortable with having you play with us."

In an eastern hospital, the vice president of human resources joined the bowling league and found that many of the employees seemed uncomfortable around him. Several of the employees later told him that he reminded them too much of work and that they would prefer that he not bowl in their league. Of course, in many organizations, senior managers and employees do mix well. The point here is that many times senior managers are mistaken in their belief that employees enjoy socializing with them. Enforced mixing and fraternizing between senior managers and employees is usually a misguided strategy.

The following protocols can help senior managers work effectively with employees.

Abandon the "Open Door" Policy

Senior managers have been taught for years that they need to make themselves available to employees. To maintain an "open door" policy, managers are taught to set aside certain times when employees may meet with them in their offices. This policy suggests that managers not insist on having employees move through levels of management; instead, employees have ready access to senior managers. An "open door" policy seemingly has become a major component of many positive employee-relations practices for management.

The "open door" policy itself is symbolic of managerial power in that it requires the employee to come to the manager, in contrast to the manager going to the employee. Although some employees may feel free to avail themselves of this opportunity, many more do not. Senior managers must not forget that most employees do not feel comfortable in the executive suite.

A logical solution to a possible "ivory tower" syndrome is Tom Peters's suggestion that one "manage by walking around" (MBWA). This is a step in the right direction but does not go far enough. MBWA typically involves a rather cursory and superficial walk-through. Employees in many organizations have come to expect and barely tolerate these tours. Senior managers can improve on this by employing the following protocols.

Leave the Office Regularly and Frequently

Senior managers and executives should get out into the organization and spend as much time as possible with the staff on their own turf. They should consider the possibility of working with certain departments or units for four-, six-, or even eight- hour periods, rotating through several departments over a period of months. One well-known CEO keeps a number of uniforms from different departments in his office and frequently dons them and goes to work with employees in different departments.

Have Lunch and Share Breaks Frequently with Employees

Health care managers and executives should spend time going in the employee cafeteria and sitting with various groups of employees. Such encounters can uncover an amazing amount of information and numerous insights.

Many senior managers pride themselves on the fact that they lunch with a selected group of employees each month to enhance communications and understanding. This is an excellent practice but should not take the place of informal opportunities to mix with employees. Although many employees enjoy these formal opportunities, others may perceive these occasions as just another free lunch for the executive.

Make Off-Shift Visits

Executives should visit the night shift at 1:00 A.M. or 2:00 A.M., not 6:00 A.M. or 7:00 A.M., when employees are at the busiest point in the shift as they prepare to go home. Executives should also consider spending an *entire* shift with the night staff. This is one way to truly get a sense of their work life.

Take Extra Time to Listen

When interacting with employees, the time spent truly listening in depth to their concerns will pay valuable dividends. Employees will often bring up issues and problems gradually over the course of the conversation, carefully checking managers' reactions. If they are interrupted too early in the process, they may never get to their real concerns. Many senior managers find themselves trying to solve specific problems, only to find out later that those were not the real problems.

Keep in mind that there will always be some real or perceived barrier between senior managers and employees. By recognizing this, one can place more emphasis on truly hearing and understanding issues and concerns.

Initiate a Job-Shadowing Program

A job-shadowing program allows an employee to spend an entire day with a senior manager as he or she works; the senior manager then spends an entire day with the employee at his or her job.

Job-shadowing programs differ from the department-rotation idea in that they are a more personalized approach dedicated to spending time with just one employee. They can also be developed in a formalized manner to enhance the understanding of a particular job or unit. Another benefit is that job-shadowing often develops "grapevine" sources of information for senior managers.

Consider the Impact of Your Behaviors

Do Not Touch Other Employees

A handshake is the only appropriate form of physical interaction in a business setting because it is least subject to misinterpretation.

Confining touching to handshakes is more than just an excellent rule to avoid sexual harassment difficulties. Many managers, particularly senior managers, tend to touch employees when offering praise or giving instruction: for example, they may offer a pat on the back or put their arm around an employee's shoulders. There are several problems with these actions. First, they suggest a parent-child relationship. The work setting should reflect an adult-adult alliance, and a suggestion of anything else is inappropriate.

Many employees feel that they are being treated like children when patted or touched in this fashion, although they may not say so. Second, these actions imply that one party, the manager, has greater power. This makes the employee feel subservient. This certainly is contrary to the popular philosophies of today's leadership, which emphasize the empowerment of employees. The last thing that senior managers should do is create feelings of inferiority through a misinterpreted touch. Such feelings could make it difficult to inspire employees to be partners with management in the mission of the organization.

Employees who are members of groups that historically have been oppressed may be particularly sensitive regarding touching that is perceived as patronizing. To prevent sending the wrong message, executives should try to become familiar with the cultures and attitudes represented within the organization. It is better not to touch at all than to risk offending an employee.

Adhering to this no-touching rule will also help senior managers avoid real or perceived sexual harassment situations. Touches carry with them all kinds of meanings, including unintended sexual suggestions. This is an area where all senior managers must exercise caution.

This protocol is simple enough, but it also leaves the manager questioning what might be done in place of the well-intentioned physical touch. People can be "touched" with a smile, a compliment, or public praise. Handwritten notes may also provide an alternative for the manager.

Before touring work areas, the senior manager should recall the image of a general's "white-glove" inspection. Too often those who are being inspected believe that the primary purpose of the visit is to find something wrong. This is not the intended message of a senior manager's visit to the "troops." Spending some extra time in the work area will go a long way toward increasing the bond between senior managers and employees.

Use Caution When Making Unplanned Comments

Senior managers and executives should choose their words carefully when they are with groups of employees, avoiding poorly thought-out comments that might be misinterpreted by the employee.

They should be equally cautious when criticizing employees. They should be careful to target the undesirable behavior, not the person. Criticism in front of others is absolutely to be avoided; it is guaranteed to bring humiliation, and today workers will not tolerate that.

Senior managers tend to give directions or orders to employees, especially during their walks around the institution. Employees often perceive such comments as criticism. One can imagine employees commenting after the senior manager provides instruction and direction: 'What would she know? How long has it been since she has done any real work?' In these situations senior managers are frequently misinterpreted when giving guidance.

Be Positive and Optimistic

This is the message of Zig Ziglar, a popular and successful motivational speaker. A chapter in Ziglar's book *See You at the Top* is entitled: "Good or Bad, You Pass It On."[1] A person's personality and character always affect others. High-energy people tend to energize those around them. Managers who show excitement when faced with challenges tend to get more effort from their staff. Those who are sullen or negative often engender negative attitudes in others. One of the worst influences within any group are the naysayers, those persons who come up with reasons why no approach to problems will work and who find fault with any situation. The ability to be positive and optimistic may be one of the most important skills any manager can possess when dealing with employees.

This protocol is actually part of good leadership discipline. Effective leaders always exhibit a positive approach and outlook. This is particularly true when they are around employees. Many managers have a tendency to act less than positive, thinking that this makes them seem more like employees. Other managers are simply unwilling to make the effort to be upbeat and positive; they are content to stay skeptical and pessimistic. Senior managers and executives must often make very deliberate voluntary efforts to be positive.

Management consultant Marilyn Moats Kennedy teaches that although managers need not always "feel" the role, they must always "act" the role. At times it is necessary and appropriate for managers to disguise certain negative feelings in order to be effective leaders.

Senior managers should examine their approaches to people and the atmosphere they create as they meet with employees. This is particularly true when they are doing such ordinary and routine things as coming in from the parking lot or picking up their lunch in the cafeteria. Many employees value these opportunities to see the senior managers and derive a certain amount of inspiration and encouragement from them. These are excellent opportunities for senior managers to generate enthusiasm for the organization and its programs.

In *Positive Management Practices*, Arthur C. Beck and Ellis D. Hillmar describe the need to have a positive attitude. "Negative energy is a depleter, causing hopelessness, helplessness, and powerlessness. With negative energy, people see no possibilities or choices; they are resistant to change and use their energy against the manager and the organization. Negative energy is soon exhausted, leaving little or no energy at all."[2]

One common element found in almost all effective managers is their positive energy. They always seem willing and anxious to challenge all problems and issues. These managers enjoy the opportunity to try every approach possible to deal with difficulties. Their positive attitude is contagious and spreads through the organization. The following protocols are effective in increasing positive energy.

Have a positive facial expression. Executives should learn to look positively positive. Their faces should show joy in being where they are. They should smile as often as possible when around other employees.

Do not complain. As was discussed in Chapter 3, leaders should not complain. They should realize that employees typically see executives as being in enviable positions and have difficulty understanding what executives have to complain about. Senior managers and executives should also realize that things could be much worse.

Bad-mouthing, making unwarranted negative comments about situations or people, can be very counterproductive. At times managers may do this to play negative politics within the office or the organization; this can have negative consequences. Senior managers should avoid making negative comments that have no constructive value.

Adopt a "can-do" attitude. This was discussed in Chapter 5 but bears repeating here. Individuals who have a "can do" attitude can break the bureaucracy and get things done.

Integrate and Support Continuous Quality Improvement

Continuous quality improvement (CQI) programs demand a lot of interaction among senior executives and other employees. Successful CQI implementation requires that senior leaders be willing and able to release some of the control they traditionally have possessed. Employees need to have the ability to work within an environment where they feel comfortable challenging processess in order to make needed improvements in quality outcomes. For CQI programs to work, the barriers between senior leadership and employees should be taken down. Senior executives should try to provide guidance and to clear the path for employees to improve their work.

Many of the suggestions in this chapter can assist senior executives with CQI in their organizations. The extra time an executive takes to listen to employees and the executive's positive and optimistic outlook on the organization are important components of a CQI initiative.

Summary

Some senior managers often take pride in their ability to deal with employees and are confident in their communication and interaction skills with all levels of employees. However, few managers would deny that there is a credibility gap between management and the employee population. This gap may be great or small, depending upon a variety of circumstances, but nonetheless exists.

It takes a great deal of effort and time to bridge the gap. Senior managers should work at managing the perceptions held by employees within their organizations. They should try to spend as much time interacting with employees as they do with medical staff and board and community leaders.

The protocols discussed in this chapter will help improve relationships between management and employees. They seem to be no more than old-fashioned common sense, but they are nonetheless important and potent. Human resources will be the most important resources in health care in the years to come. Managers should make serious efforts to enhance and strengthen their abilities to work with employees.

Notes

1. Z. Ziglar, *See You at the Top* (New York: Pelican Publishing Company, 1977), 118.
2. A. C. Beck and E. D. Hillmar, *Positive Management Practices* (San Francisco: Jossey-Bass, 1986), 67.

9

Protocols for Working
with Other Executives

This chapter is directed at vice presidents, assistant and associate administrators, and other senior managers. It is crucial that these executives work together as harmoniously as possible, especially as competition in health care grows more intense.

The growing number of health care administrators in the labor market has increased internal competitiveness. However, attempts to undercut others to enhance one's own career almost always harm organizational success and the success of the health care executive.

It is human nature for those competing for scarce resources and the time and attention of others to be selfish. Most people want to receive their share of honor and recognition and will compete vigorously to get it. However, minimizing selfish, competitive behavior *can* prove to be rewarding to one's career and to the organization. The key to success rests in top management's ability to assemble a group of senior-level managers who are willing to minimize their personal interests for the good of the management team. This requires a strong top manager who is able to elicit the altruistic characteristics of each senior manager.

The protocols described in this chapter are intended to improve relationships among members of the senior management team and thereby increase the success of the team.

Common Causes of Team Friction

Before outlining the protocols, it is useful to consider two common causes of team friction and poor interaction: jealousy and envy, and tunnel vision.

These all-too-human shortcomings, if uncontrolled, can be quite destructive to an organization and its team-building efforts.

Jealousy and Envy

Jealousy can exist when there is an unhealthy rivalry or competition between individuals; it frequently appears when people perceive that there are unequal standards for gaining recognition and rewards. In health care organizations, reporting relationships are a frequent cause of jealousy. In some organizations, some vice presidents report to the chief operating officer, whereas other vice presidents report to the chief executive officer. This differentiation among vice presidents can lead to jealousy on the part of those vice presidents who report to the chief operating officer, who is lower in the organizational hierarchy than the chief executive officer. Thus, it is problematic to have a senior team that has two levels of reporting relationships. Difficulties also become more acute when senior managers are closely aligned with a particular area of expertise. In some cases, the chief financial officer reports to the chief executive officer and the chief marketing officer reports to the chief operating officer. Other examples include having a chief nursing officer report to a senior operations officer, whereas chief officers in other disciplines report directly to the chief executive officer. These problem situations have increased over the past decade with the growth in the number of multicorporate arrangements. There are occasions when simply calling certain positions "senior vice president" instead of "vice president" has caused friction and strife.

A similar situation exists when other vice presidents become jealous of the vice president of nursing within organizations because they believe that nursing receives the bulk of organizational resources. These peers may believe that the nursing vice president enjoys an advantage as a result. This jealousy often surfaces in discussions pertaining to budgets and staffing. What the other vice presidents often fail to take into account, however, is that nursing is the area in which most patient complaints surface and in which physicians demand the most support and resources. Nursing executives must help their peers understand this but also must participate as total team players when cuts must be made.

Organizations can also have problems when other officers are jealous of chief financial officers because they control the organizational purse strings. Such jealousy can be very damaging to the overall team effort and, ultimately, organizational success.

Jealousy can also exist between senior managers in staff and line positions. The staff managers often believe that they are subordinate to the line managers. As a result, they create control mechanisms within their areas of responsibility to increase their influence. To avoid this damaging jealousy, both groups have to develop an enhanced understanding of role. Senior managers in staff positions must work hard not to create bureaucratic obstacles for managers in line positions.

One suggestion for minimizing the negative effects of jealousy is to create an environment in which all senior managers fully understand and appreciate one another's role. One way to accomplish this is to have all senior management officers take administrative call (rather than just the line executives) and ensure that all make executive rounds. By doing this, staff executives will gain an increased understanding of line issues.

Another suggestion is to have a staff executive cover for a line executive who is on vacation, and vice versa. For example, the vice president of marketing serves as the backup for the vice president of professional and clinical services, and vice versa; the vice president of finance is the backup for the vice president of nursing, and vice versa. During vacations, the backup would literally occupy the other's office for a period of time, hold the regular meetings of that division, and supervise the managers of the area. One chief executive officer who had his team do this found that the pairs of executives became much closer organizationally and worked better together as a team.

Many problems in senior management teams are also caused by the desire to have more power or authority or departments. Of course, a certain amount of this acquisitive attitude gives managers the drive to aspire to more responsible executive positions. This attitude can be negative, however, if it is not placed in proper perspective. That perspective requires a team orientation and a willingness to compromise on issues for the greater good of the team.

Envy is a resentment and coveting of others' resources or talents. It can be quite destructive to a senior team. Covetousness causes people to want what others have (material and tangible objects as well as intangibles such as charisma and technical skill) so badly that it overtakes all other activities.

Senior managers can covet, among other things

- space (personal office or departmental);
- staff (e.g., FTEs);
- access to the CEO (reporting relationship or nearby office);
- access to the board (attendance at board meetings);
- time with the CEO;
- equipment (e.g., car phone and home fax machine);
- responsibility and authority;

- departments and cost centers;
- capital equipment (e.g., larger, newer, and more sophisticated computers); and
- information.

Unfortunately, due to cost and space considerations, executive suites cannot be designed so that all of the offices are the same size, all of the telephones contain the same speaker phone devices, and so on. With the right leadership, senior-level managers will focus more on organizational goals and less on executive offices.

All people are envious at times; however, when envy becomes extreme and all-consuming it jeopardizes the team atmosphere. Furthermore, it isolates senior managers from others and decreases sharing of information and resources, all of which are detrimental to the team, the individual managers, and the organization.

Tunnel Vision

Senior-level executives in health care are no more immune to tunnel vision than are senior-level executives in other industries. Tunnel vision is the tendency to view only a single dimension of an organization or to consider only one point of view or to view one's areas of responsibilities as more important than any other areas. In fact, one might argue that the high degree of specialization of most senior-level managers in health care makes them especially prone to tunnel vision. Many (especially chief nursing officers) have come up through the ranks via a specialist track. Other than those who have been line administrators, true generalists in health care are rare. Even in those cases, line administrators rarely have staff experience in human resources, marketing, or finance.

Tunnel vision can result in problems in situations with high-stakes payoffs and penalties. In these cases, senior managers with tunnel vision typically retreat to their own areas of expertise and identify problems and possible solutions from that single perspective.

For example, if an organization faces serious financial difficulties and must institute across-the-board budget cuts, many senior executives will do anything possible to protect their own areas. This is not always done for selfish reasons but often because the tunnel vision of managers who are primarily specialists prevents them from seeing the bigger organizational picture.

One nursing executive in a major teaching hospital customarily kept large numbers of budgeted vacancies in the nursing labor expense budget so that she could overhire additional nurses whenever experienced nurses applied at the medical center. During the 1980s, when there were increasing needs to reduce expenses, this institution went through several attrition-reduction programs and eliminated a number of vacant lines. This nursing executive was able to cut several full-time employees (FTEs) without incurring any inconvenience. This tunnel-vision approach was very detrimental to team effectiveness in this situation.

Problems arise when executives believe that the solution falls only under their jurisdiction. For example, many human resources executives believe that compensation issues fall exclusively in their domain. They will constantly take charge of the overall compensation program and often, as a result, get little buy-in from other executives when changes in the pay program are made. Other senior managers also find it easy to pass the blame on to human resources if there are problems.

Budgets and fiscal responsibility provide another example. Often line managers pass much of the burden and blame to fiscal services during budget problems.

Tunnel vision often develops when there are few opportunities for meaningful sharing of information among members of the senior team. Senior teams are often so busy that each individual member focuses upon his or her own particular areas and there is little time for cross-sharing of information and ideas. It is then difficult to get team members to focus on issues that do not directly and immediately affect them.

Managers also develop tunnel vision when a decision seems to affect only a limited area. Often, they do not carefully consider the ripple effect of such decisions and pay little attention to issues that seemingly do not pertain to their areas of responsibility.

A number of years ago, Bernard Lachner, president of Evanston Hospital Corporation, was asked to address a national association meeting of human resources executives in health care. He was to answer the question: "Should human resources be a part of senior management?" His answer was in the form of a question: "What does the chief human resources officer bring to the table?" If the only element that the chief human resources officer brought was the human resources perspective, Lachner felt that he or she should not be a part of the senior management team. He expected all of his senior executives to bring a much broader perspective to the decision-making process.

Michael H. Covert, another health care executive, told his senior team that he expected them to act as though they were chief operating officers when they sat at the administrative table. He asked his administrative staff to represent their own areas of responsibility but to take on a broader perspective when the time came to make decisions as a team.

Obstacles to Senior-Level Teamwork

Many senior managers do not like team-building exercises or management development programs that attempt to improve how the executive team works together. They may consider this type of behavior soft and intangible. They may not wish to recognize their own limitations. Many will not spend time listening to suggestions and solutions for team enhancement. Some senior managers rarely go to management development programs and may feel that attendance at their own in-house programs is a sign of weakness. Finally, some teams are already at such a heightened competitive level that appropriate teamwork is not possible. In these situations, it may be necessary to utilize routine team meetings as efforts turn toward team building.

Elements of Teamwork

There are several main elements of teamwork that need to be understood to ensure good teamwork. These elements are especially important for senior-level management teams. The sections below discuss the key elements: the group process, information sharing, group norms and enforcement, cohesiveness, and conflict management.

The Group Process

The group process is the most important element of teamwork. It is the methods whereby team members give and take and engage in prioritizing activities and group problem solving. Senior executives must understand how each group functions. They must understand the principles involved in how groups come together and select their leaders. They must have a clear understanding of how information is processed and decisions are made. They must have a full awareness of how group members censure one another and apply sanctions. Finally, they must realize that how they approach different groups and apply group processes will reflect on them.

In team building there are four success factors. All four factors should be present to achieve an effective group process. These four factors are:

1. The group must have a set of common goals. As senior management candidates consider joining other organizations, they should seriously consider their compatibility with the goals of the existing team and how those teams work together toward those goals.

2. Group members should be on an equal footing. A lack of parity causes deep psychological divisions that may not surface until the team faces tough challenges.
3. The group leader must draw out the opinions of all of the members and ensure that every viewpoint is given equal consideration.
4. There must be some degree of mutual dependence among group members.

The fourth factor is perhaps the most important in team building.

Group Norms and Enforcement

The establishment and enforcement of group norms are crucial to the group process and the success of team-building efforts. A norm is an attitude or a set of unwritten rules that govern the behavior and outlook of a group. Senior management teams have group norms, just as lower-level workers do, but they often enforce conformity in more ruthless ways, by failing to cooperate or by cutting off information, because senior management group members have greater power and control over resources and information. Also, the consequences of being a renegade in a group of senior managers are greater than in work groups at other levels within the organization because the need for shared information is greater and because more senior-level managers can have more influence in negating another team member's effectiveness.

Conformity to group norms is crucial to executive cooperation. Members who do not conform disrupt the effectiveness of team operations. Because groups quickly develop their norms and maintain them rather rigidly over time, many new chief executive officers believe that they must clean house to derive new norms to move the organization in the desired direction.

Cohesiveness

The cohesiveness of team members is important to good teamwork. Keeping the size of the group small and all members on equal footing will enhance cohesiveness. As an example, too many organizations are so layered with titles of different rank and status (such as senior vice president as well as vice president) that it can be difficult to achieve this cohesion.

Conflict Management

There is no more crucial issue in teamwork than the ability to manage and resolve conflict. It is often unlikely that the conflict that arises within a senior team can be resolved; rather, the best hope often is to manage it. Conflict resolution techniques strive to eliminate the sources of conflict, whereas conflict management techniques recognize that although these sources may always be present, they can be minimized (managed) so that the outcome fits within the overall goals of the organization. The concept of "fighting fair," discussed later in this chapter, is an important tool for conflict management. There are several guiding principles of conflict management.

Conflict management is complex. Conflict does not occur in a simplistic world; there rarely is only *one* cause of conflict. Although there may be only one surface issue, conflict usually takes place against a more complex backdrop. The struggle over a single issue is a smokescreen for deeper friction over such issues as power, ego, authority, and pride.

Conflict management is more than just a win-or-lose situation. Although in conflict situations there may be a single issue that can be "won" or "lost," often there are deeper issues involved in the controversy. Most participants are willing to lose some battles in hopes of winning the war. To put conflict management in win-lose terminology is to turn it into a single sports-type game. Organizational life is certainly not that. On many occasions, both parties must give in, and as a result, both lose part of their original position.

Remember the relationship. Instead of approaching conflict from a win-lose perspective, senior managers should keep in mind that the relationship with the other person(s) is ultimately more important than the actual conflict situation. This forms the foundation for compromise.

Compromise. Compromise is not negative behavior; it is appropriate in team situations. Senior managers who can compromise and thus work well with fellow team members will find that their individual effectiveness is enhanced. Their willingness to compromise and not view each encounter as a life-or-death challenge will make others more willing to aid and compromise with them. Often, the art of compromise involves identifying other issues of importance. The ability to trade one issue for another forms the framework for conflict management.

The classic example of compromise is the typical labor negotiation. When unions and management negotiate, they try to package issues together and make trades so that both parties go away from the interaction with some wins and some losses. A conflict on a single issue is difficult to manage. Successful conflict management strives to provide several issues to ponder within the framework of the discussion.

Clarify Authority and Accountability

Senior managers should work very hard together to eliminate any unclear job responsibilities or areas that could create conflict. Senior management teams should devote time at least once a year to addressing and clarifying organizational lines of influence and authority. There should be regular and open discussions of areas of responsibility and accountability. These deliberations should be part of a formal annual organizational audit process.

Have a Strong Team Leader

A strong team will have a strong leader and congruity on mission and goals. It is only with these characteristics that a team can be strong and cooperative.

Building the Capacity for Effective
Senior-Level Teamwork

The type of organization affects its capacity for teamwork. Many of the protocols described below suggest attitudes and behaviors that could be personally counterproductive for an individual senior manager. For example, they would not be effective in an organization with an already intensely negative competitive spirit among senior managers. The organization that has a CEO who leads by divisiveness is not one that will be open to the recommended organizational behavior practices. If the reader works in an organization that values intrigue and destructive group behavior, these protocols will certainly not be helpful. In this type of situation, it may be best to seek other employment.

The following protocols are designed to improve interaction and teamwork among senior-level managers and thus increase the overall effectiveness of the organization.

Share Information

Members of the senior management team must be committed to sharing information. Many books describe how to build sources of power and develop areas of influence by withholding information and doling it out as a return for a favor. This is not ideal for executive growth in that it jeopardizes senior-level teamwork.

Competent senior managers and executives should be confident enough to share information appropriately at all times. They should know that sharing information will actually assist them in the pursuit of their goals because one must share information to get it.

Encourage Healthy Conflict

Fellow executives should disagree often! Conflicts are very natural out-growths of interpersonal situations. However, as we discussed earlier, senior-level conflicts are often *managed* rather than *resolved*. Healthy controversy and confrontation should be encouraged, not repressed. In doing so, the concerns causing conflict can at least be surfaced. Unfortunately, our society does not teach conflict management skills and discourages conflict between children both at home and in schools. The ability to get along with others usually means not fighting or arguing with them. Senior managers must stimulate healthy conflict, conflict that is handled in a professional and team-spirited manner. The following guidelines contribute to healthy conflict.

Fight fair. When senior managers fight, they should fight fair. There are several rules for a fair fight. They are:

Fight based upon facts, not emotions. Health care executives frequently must deal with emotionally charged issues, arguments and defenses. The following statements are often heard:

- "If you do not do this, our patients will suffer."
- "We cannot deliver the services you are asking for."
- "We have given tons of justification for our request."
- "Our staff are the ones who collect the money—without them, we could not stay in business."
- "The acuity is just going higher and higher."
- "These patients are sicker than the ones last year."

In a fair fight, the adversaries present true and appropriate facts about the dispute. Each allows the other side to challenge the validity of those facts and present counterpoints. The adversaries are open to appropriate challenges of their facts and are willing to accept correction when relevant.

Listen to the opposition. Adversaries should give fair consideration to their opponent's points. This requires restraint and open-mindedness and is abso-lutely necessary for the good of the overall team.

Do not gunny-sack. "Gunny-sacking" means raising a barrage of past argu-ments and attempting to blast the opposition with these no-longer-relevant issues. Another form of gunny-sacking is bringing up past problems that were solved because of one person's willingness to compromise. The gunny-sacker is quick to remind everyone of their past sacrifices. In doing so, they are trying to gain concessions from others because they have supposedly already made their own concessions.

Do not turtle. This is sometimes called the silent technique. A turtler does not do much debating but instead remains quiet. Often, this person will wait until later and sabotage any agreement reached or distort the true arrangements on the outcome of the controversy. It is at this later point in time that they finally raise their points and suggest that not all issues were fully considered in the argument.

Argue the issue, not the personalities or the environment. Senior managers should not say, for example, "Well, you are in nursing, and nursing always gets what it wants whether right or wrong." Nor should they say something like, "You never contribute because you are so selfish."

Be assertive, not aggressive. Present the points within the context of a debate, not in a combative fashion.

Fight soon. Air your disagreements sooner rather than later. Do not allow issues to simmer below the surface.

Be prepared to compromise. This is essential. When the conflict is over and there is an agreement, repeat the terms and conditions of the agreement once again before ending the session.

Recognize Formal and Informal Team Roles

Senior executives should recognize the informal roles that each team member plays within a group. They should remember that each member of a team brings different expertise and skills to the group. Some serve as facilitators, for example, others are rulekeepers who ensure that fights are fought fairly, and still others serve as informal arbitrators who announce and enforce decisions when compromise is not possible.

Establish Accountability

Accountability—the assignment of responsibility—is essential for successful group efforts. The main purpose of accountability is to ensure that something gets done. As teams work together, there are two potential conflicts over accountability. The first results when senior managers all *want* responsibility for an area or function; the other results when senior managers all *do not want* responsibility for an area or function. It is critical that a CEO or COO clearly delineate organizational structure and the rationale behind why accountability is assigned as it is.

In health care organizations, unclear guidelines on decision-making and signing authority often create conflict at all levels of the organization about who is responsible for performing certain functions. Often these problems are solved on a one-to-one basis between employees. Sometimes, however, more serious conflicts are pushed up within the organizational hierarchy and end up with senior managers.

Organizational charts are drawn in part to avoid some of this conflict, but they are not the complete answer. Most solutions take the aggressive sponsorship of the CEO or other governing head in clarifying responsibilities, in setting forth clear lines of authority, and in spending frequent time discussing potentially overlapping responsibilities.

Summary

How senior managers work with one another determines an organization's success; as the team goes, so typically goes the organization. Unfortunately, selfishness and desire for personal power, influence, and rewards can sabotage effective team work. The protocols discussed in this chapter help senior managers to set aside negative feelings and behavior, and to contribute to effective team interaction. Often, the successes that teams may achieve are tied to the guidance and direction of the CEO.

10

PROTOCOLS FOR WORKING
WITH THE BOARD OF TRUSTEES

This chapter is targeted primarily at the CEO of an organization, who is the person who most frequently works with a board of trustees. These are, however, protocols that are quite useful to all senior executives. Many senior managers aspire toward CEO positions in which they will need to interact with a board of trustees. Relationships with the board are often as critical to the success of a health care CEO as those with the medical staff. Mistakes can be disastrous.

Reponsibilities of the Board of Trustees
of a Health Care Organization

Within the legal framework of the corporate entity, the governing board of a health care organization has the ultimate legal and fiscal responsibility for the organization's operations. Courts of law, government regulatory agencies, and the Joint Commission on the Accreditation of Healthcare Organizations (JCAHO) all look to the governing board as the final authority for the health care corporation.

Governing boards have several basic responsibilities. One is described in legal terms as "preserving the institution's assets." A board does this by (a) monitoring the organization's financial condition; (b) having oversight authority over the organization's entering into contracts; (c) ensuring that there is adequate business and liability insurance coverage; (d) monitoring and guiding the organization through any legal suits; and (e) supervising the collection of revenues. In summary, the board attempts to ensure that the organization is managed in accordance with sound business principles.

Most boards perform these functions through committees that oversee the actions taken by the organization's management. For example, financial activity is reviewed by the board's finance committee.

A second responsibility of the board is to ensure the provision of adequate and competent patient care. The courts (and the JCAHO) have continued to hold that boards must ensure the competency of caregivers (particularly the medical staff). The board must establish mechanisms for reviewing credentials prior to granting practice privileges to physicians and institute methods to review the quality of care given in the organization.

A third responsibility of a board of trustees is the selection of the corporation's chief executive officer. This, of course, is one of the more important responsibilities of a board and is often a major area of conflict among board members as they select and work with CEOs.

Finally, emanating from the board's responsibilities is a legal liability called a fiduciary liability. This means that something (such as a corporation) is placed in the trust of or care of a person or persons who serve as fiduciaries who hold the highest degree of liability for acts and omissions of acts of a corporation. As a result, members of boards of trustees of health care organizations take on a very serious responsibility.

The above discussion provides a context for understanding the issues surrounding relationships with boards of trustees. The protocols discussed in this chapter are important because most board members (understandably) take their responsibility very seriously. They are fully aware of their fiduciary liability and are committed to fulfilling their obligations to the organization regardless of the potential liability.

Protocols for Smooth Relations with Boards of Trustees

CEOs can find their continued employment in jeopardy because of poor relationships with their board members. Sometimes difficult situations are purely political; many other times, however, they are the result of board members' concern about the organization. The protocols discussed below can help CEOs and senior managers and executives work well with their boards.

Participate in the Screening of Board Members

CEOs should try to be involved as much as possible in the screening of prospective members. They should meet with each prospect and describe the time commitments required by board membership and board members' obligations. By giving prospective board members a true sense of the health care industry, its peculiarities, and its special challenges, health care CEOs can help to ensure that they will understand the issues and concerns. Finally, when meeting with prospective board members, CEOs should try to get the prospect to make a true commitment to serve.

Board membership in health care organizations is no longer an honorary position. It should not be a reward for those who give significant amounts of money to the organization. It is a time-consuming and challenging job, and board members need to be willing and prepared to spend time in orientation, both to the health care field and to the individual organization. During the screening interview, CEOs should delineate the key issues for health care in general and the institution in particular. CEOs should try to ascertain that prospects understand the complexity and difficulties facing the organization.

Prepare for Conflicts of Interest

Make provisions for dealing with board members' conflicts of interest. Typically, written statements identify potential sources of conflict of interest such as business dealings with the corporation. These statements are designed to help guard against board members taking advantage of their position on the board for personal gain. The key here is to identify potential areas of conflict of interest. There is no guarantee that board members will not use their positions for personal gain. It is helpful, however, to have all the existing relationships spelled out for the entire board to see.

Board members who are also physicians can present a difficult situation. Although it is beneficial to have physician representation on the board of directors, obviously board members who are members of the medical staff will always have a relationship with the corporation. Frequently, they are very active, influential members of the medical staff and are financially valuable to the organization in that they admit a large number of patients. Also, they often are extremely loyal to the organization. All of these factors can cause other board members to overlook positions taken by physician members, claiming conflicts of interest. This is an area fraught with potential problems. There should be a clearly written and frequently discussed conflict-of-interest provision that requires physician board members to remove themselves from any deliberations or actions that directly affect them as members of the medical staff.

Communicate

CEOs should avoid presenting board members with surprises. If at all possible, CEOs should notify them in advance of any potentially damaging news stories or other adverse situations. Fax or send by messenger any negative reports or stories so that board members do not find out about them by chance—or from outsiders. Mechanisms should be in place to guarantee an adequate flow of information. CEOs should also have in place a specific plan for communicating with board members in the event of a crisis.

CEOs should be certain to contact board members about problems, concerns, and issues. One CEO of a southern hospital visited each board member once a month to touch base and briefly cover the agenda of the upcoming board meeting. By doing this, she not only communicated board issues but also developed a better personal working relationship with each member.

In working with a board, senior executives should guard against communicating primarily with just one member or a small group of members. Often, this occurs when CEOs work primarily with board executive committees. Board members who are not members of executive committees may feel left out of the decision-making process. A number of CEOs have discovered much too late that board members had taken offense at this seeming exclusion by the CEO and took action against him or her.

Learn How to Manage Controversy

Often controversial issues will surface in the course of a meeting. Ideally, discussion on these controversial issues should be postponed until later board meetings to allow time for consensus building and to determine where members stand on the issues. It is best that the board deal with tough issues only after thorough preparation. Executives should work hard with the board officers to keep items that are not on the agenda out of the discussion.

However, controversy cannot be put off forever. Difficult issues must be raised and addressed. As was discussed in Chapter 2, there is merit in putting everything on the table. Executives should protect their credibility by being as open and honest as possible with board members and should not try to hide things from them.

Respect Board Members' Time and Schedules

As busy as health care CEOs are, they should remember that board members are also busy. The time they commit to board membership is taken from their own professions and families. For self-employed persons, such as attorneys, time spent away from their practices doing hospital board work is money out of their pockets.

Meetings should start on time and should run as efficiently as possible. There is no possible excuse for CEOs or other members of the administrative staff being tardy. Many successful CEOs arrange with their board chairs to set time allocations for each item on the board agenda. Many will also put this time allocation on the agenda itself. Thus, each presenter and each board member knows in advance the time allotted for each topic.

CEOs should be certain to send relevant materials to all board members far enough in advance for them to have time to review it. The material should be comprehensive and free of errors. (Although everyone makes mistakes, CEOs must allow *no* mistakes in material sent to the board.) Each article should, when at all possible, have a summary attached to it so that the members can quickly grasp each issue before exploring the detail.

Whenever possible individual meetings with board members should be held at their places of business. This shows them the ultimate in respect and consideration of their time. Also, board members often will feel more comfortable meeting off-site and will accomplish more. Off-site visits usually minimize interruptions and will provide the CEO with an opportunity to see members' places of business. When board members visit the health care organization, the CEO and executives should see them promptly and offer as much hospitality as possible. Although it would seem to go without saying, the CEO should remind the secretarial and support staff who greet board members of the importance of respecting members' time, talents, and willingness to serve.

Provide Ongoing Education

Regular and meaningful ongoing education of board members can be an important way to develop and maintain positive relationships. Many problems are caused by simple deficiencies in knowledge. Unfortunately, many boards do not take the time for regular education and development. CEOs can start an education program by offering a detailed and meaningful orientation to new board members. Too often, it is mistakenly assumed that meaningful board education must involve outside speakers and formal retreats at getaway locations. However, many boards have successfully implemented ongoing education by devoting a thirty-minute period at the beginning of each meeting to in-depth coverage of a specific topic. The more board members know about the health care field, the organization, and the issues confronting the organization, the better able they will be to support the CEO and his or her policies.

Coordinate All Communication through the CEO

CEOs should be certain that their key staff members understand that the CEO is the main contact with the board members and that all of their work needs to be channeled through the CEO. Often, some senior managers will work so closely with board committees that they will attempt to deal directly with board members and problems result. These senior managers may second-guess the CEO's decisions or undermine the CEO by giving information inappropriately to board members. This is particularly true for the chief financial officer or the vice president of medical affairs. Coordination is necessary to set priorities and avoid conflicts. It is crucial that senior management present a united front on common issues. Also, the CEO should closely monitor any work the staff does with various board committees to ensure its quality and completeness.

Understand Board Members' Community Roles

CEOs and other senior executives should be aware of the other community activities of board members. It may be good "public relations" for health care executives to contribute their own time (and perhaps money) to issues that are important to their board members. For example, if a board member is chair of the local community fund drive, the organization should participate in the drive.

Be Positive about the Organization's Past Leadership

Senior executives should never cast any negative light on their predecessor(s). CEOs, particularly those who have been brought in to accomplish a turn-around, should never make negative comments about the efforts and results of the past administration. They should remember that some (or all) of the current board members may believe that the comments on the past administration cast a negative reflection on them. Board members may also feel that the negative statements about past leadership are being made to enhance present achievements. Present leaders should let their accomplishments speak for themselves. If executives receive praise for their work that is accompanied by negative comments about the past administration, the executive should accept the compliments gratefully and ignore the criticism of past leadership.

Maintain Decorum

During meetings with individual board members and the full board, executives should maintain a serious atmosphere, in keeping with the nature of the issues with which these bodies deal as well as the board's fiduciary relationship to the organization.

A CEO encountered problems with his board when a well-known planning consultant presented a proposal during which he, while discussing pricing strategies for mammography services and the full OB/GYN product line, made several joking references to "lettuce and tomatoes" and how they related to "salad dressing." One board member had just had a mastectomy and took great offense at the light-hearted presentation of such serious issues. Several other board members resented the "humorous" approach to planning. The board refused to allow the consultant to work with the institution, even though the CEO wanted him. Worse yet, the CEO lost a great deal of credibility with the board.

In another example, a human resources consultant who was updating a board on labor issues in health care made some seemingly innocent jokes about unions. The remarks offended a member who was related to a union leader and another member whose company had very good relations with unions and felt that it was totally inappropriate to put unions down through caustic humor.

In yet another example, a marketing consultant lost business during his presentation to the board by telling "doctor" jokes and referring to the need to "take docs by the hand and lead them." The physicians on the board did not find these remarks funny.

Avoid Hiring Relatives of Board Members

Generally speaking, CEOs should not hire relatives of board members. There are too many possibilities for problems, ranging from charges of favoritism to the need to terminate a board member's relative who is not suited for a position.

Of course, there can be several mitigating factors. First, there may be a long organizational history of hiring members' relatives that cannot be ended abruptly—or at all. Second, the organization may be located in a community where such hiring is an expected practice and occurs in most other local organizations. Finally, the organization may be in a small community where the only qualified person for a job is a board member's relative. Of course, there are differences between permanent and temporary positions. The latter could possibly be filled with the relatives of board members on a short-term basis with no negative effects. However, any hiring of board members' relatives should be done only with great caution and planning.

Summary

Working well with boards is more of an art rather than a science. The art involved usually requires the application of common sense. CEOs and senior managers must always treat each board member with the utmost respect. Many problems with boards of directors result from poor or incomplete planning and faulty communication.

11

Protocols for Working
with Physicians

Before deciding that working with physicians is a rather difficult assignment, consider these facts:

- "Pre-meds" spent extra time as undergraduates in biology and chemistry labs (perhaps while business administration majors were enjoying college life)
- Medical students spent four years in "graduate" school to the MHA/MBA's two and the lawyer's three
- Physicians spend an additional one to six years in residencies or fellowships or both
- The cost of a complete medical education exceeds that of almost any other profession
- Physicians typically work ninety to one hundred hours per week during the early parts of their career
- Physicians often sacrifice more time with their families than do other career professionals
- Physicians are taught in an environment in which humiliation, challenges, and rites of passage are givens
- Physicians face constant ethical dilemmas and challenges
- Physicians serve a constituency that expects total satisfaction—a cure—and has no forgiveness or tolerance for error
- Physicians' mistakes can be fatal and even one professional mistake can end their career (or seriously harm it)
- Physicians, unlike administrators, are personally liable for professional mishaps

This list is not intended to elevate physicians over other professions. However, it is intended to help provide a context for this chapter. The professional demands upon physicians and the rigors they have endured to become physicians affect how senior managers and executives should behave toward them.

This chapter is intended to help senior managers and executives understand some of the typical demands and behaviors of physicians. Mutual respect and understanding are the keys to developing an effective working relationship between physicians and administration. In fact, some writers have suggested that future health care organizations will see increasing numbers of executives who are also physicians.

Despite the logical argument for holding physicians in high esteem, many health care administrators feel negative toward medical staff members and feel that working with them is the most difficult part of their jobs. Others believe that most physicians are so intent on their own issues and concerns that they cannot be open-minded about administrative restrictions. This attitude is not only inappropriate, it also practically guarantees that the executive will fail to develop a good working relationship with the medical staff. Physicians, given appropriate and well-reasoned information, can and do work well with administrators. The protocols described below will assist in developing good relations with the medical staff.

Effective Protocols for Working with Physicians

Senior managers most often fail to develop good working relationships with physicians because of faulty interpersonal protocols. Physicians are the gatekeepers of the health care industry as well as its most important customers. They generate most of the outcomes in the health care environment, and the public equates physicians with health care.

Health care managers should neither fear nor revere physicians—they should respect them for what they do and be given understanding of the enormous stress that society places upon them. Successful health care administrators usually have excellent personal relationships with members of the medical staff because of their sense of the appropriate. The protocols described below will enhance a sense of the appropriate in dealing with physicians.

Remember That Most Doctors Are
Self-Employed Businesspeople

Senior managers should respect physicians as independent businesspeople. They should understand how physicians' income is earned and realize that their hours are important to revenue production. (This is *not* true of most health care executives, who are salaried.) Health care executives should use caution when scheduling meetings involving physicians and be certain that those meetings start and end on time. They should also not schedule an excessive number of meetings, and those scheduled should be done so at convenient times for physicians. This respect for physicians' time will go a long way toward fostering good relationships with them.

Accept Physicians as Patient Advocates

Most physicians are the ultimate patient advocates. Organizational managers are often uncomfortable with advocates of any kind. To them, advocates push causes and issues further than they would like. Physicians must do this because of the physician-patient relationship and its obligations. Senior managers who work with doctors should be prepared to deal with advocacy issues.

Be Prepared to Give Reasons and Explanations

Health care administrators should be prepared to give *reasons* for every decision and action. To gain physician support, every policy and procedure should have a well-thought-out underlying rationale. Physicians expect this because they are trained to question every piece of information. They do this not just to challenge administrative authority but to better understand decisions and actions.

Do Not Play Favorites

Showing favoritism toward one physician or group of physicians is a quick way to harm all past efforts toward working with the medical staff. This does not mean that executives should not view key admitters differently but simply that there should always be fairness in administrative matters. Physicians who split their admissions between hospitals should be considered opportunities to increase admissions. Sometimes a little more attention and care from administrators will cause these physicians to increase admissions.

Fairness can be a problem issue in institutions with a large number of hospital-based physicians. In these situations community-based doctors frequently feel like second-class citizens. Hospital-based physicians often have more information and more frequent access to administration than do community doctors. Administrators should exercise extra care to avoid the perception that hospital-based doctors are given preference.

Provide Procedural Justice

Procedural justice is a system whereby individuals can question the reason and rationale behind actions that affect them. It allows them to challenge actions and receive an explanation. Ideally, some method of procedural justice should exist for the medical staff so that they can deal effectively with administrative issues. This system is not the formal mechanism within the medical staff bylaws that deals with credentialing and other medical staff issues. Instead, it is a method for dealing with concerns of an administrative nature (physician facilities, support of programs, capital equipment, medical record support, and the like). The procedural justice system may be rather informal; senior administrators may just need to show a willingness to hear medical staff concerns and explain their rationale for decisions.

Most physicians recognize that the concept of procedural justice does not mean that they will always get the answer or outcome they desire. They do expect, however, that they will receive a reasonable explanation. Procedural justice provides a mechanical method of appeal to the interested stakeholder (in this case, the physician). It also provides a mechanism to help physicians understand the thought processes behind administrative decisions.

Communicate, Communicate, Communicate

Physicians frequently complain that health care administrators do not keep them informed. The physician leadership should be kept apprised of events and plans. Physician leaders are not just the members of the medical executive committee or department heads; they are also the many informal leaders among the medical staff. All should be involved in the strategic planning process in a real and continuous way. The organization should have a well-written and frequently published physician newsletter. However, written communications are not always read. Senior managers should telephone physicians on a regular basis to stay in touch. Many CEOs and senior health administrators make a practice of touching base with physicians over breakfast meetings. Others have found that the golf course or the fitness club are excellent places to discuss problems and concerns and share ideas with the medical staff.

In his book, *Managing Doctors*, Dr. Alan Sheldon states: "If physicians are represented on the board, if they sit on the major committees and management sits on theirs, if management is open to physician influence and accessible, in short, if they are *involved*, then physicians usually feel positive about the appropriateness and extent of their voice."[1]

Do Not Make Clinical Decisions

Health care executives should not intervene in clearly clinical decisions. Physicians understandably become very concerned when administrators seem to try to practice medicine. Often, other physicians can be approached for suggestions as to how to address clinical problems.

Many successful executives use their medical executive committees to deal with these concerns. A full-time physician executive is a natural bridge in these matters. If at all feasible, executives should try to have a paid physician staff member who has full authority over medical staff issues. This person can intervene in situations where other physicians may raise the practice-of-medicine issue.

Identify and Address Physicians' Needs

Successful health care executives typically spend time determining and providing what the physicians in their institutions want most from the administration. Admitting physicians are actually customers and view senior administrators as the people who can effectively supply "customer service"; that is, address their needs and wants. Administrators should stay informed of what other organizations offer their medical staff and try to provide the same services and benefits. They should give physicians up-to-date, clear, concise information about their institution. They should remember that physicians' needs and wants are not always related to equipment or physical working conditions. Instead, they are often very interested in the strategic direction of the organization or in particular areas of emphasis and change.

Maintain a Physician Relations Liaison

All but the smallest hospitals should be able to afford to employ a physician relations liaison, and large hospitals should have a staff. The physician relations liaison focuses on the physicians' office staff and "small" issues and concerns that often become major sources of dissatisfaction for the medical staff. The primary job of the physician liaison is the identification and alleviation of concerns before they become large issues. The liaison must have access to the organizations' decision makers and must be able to effect change. This may seem to be an organizational issue, but it reflects on individual executives. The liaisons should be available to physicians' office staff on a routine basis.

Survey Physicians

Many successful executives survey physicians on a regular basis to determine their concerns and interests. Either written or focus group surveys can be used to identify issues of importance to the medical staff. Once identified, executives should address them as soon as is practical. This will improve physician satisfaction and enhance personal relationships between executives and physicians.

Follow Up, Follow Up, Follow Up

One of the quickest ways to lose administrative credibility is to neglect to follow up on an issue on which physicians ask for assistance or information. Senior managers and executives should keep careful track of such requests. It is dangerous to procrastinate on providing replies to physicians. They should follow up with a physician even when they must give what is, from the physician's perspective, a negative answer. And when they must give a negative answer, they should do so quickly and provide the rationale behind it. If possible, managers should consider ways to provide the physician some satisfaction through a negotiated response.

Consider Physicians' Support Staff Members

Senior managers and executives should remember the importance of the staff working for the physician. They should give staff as much organizational consideration as possible (e.g., they should be included in hospital educational programs or mailings). Most physicians utilize their staff to an even greater degree than other professions and give them much latitude and autonomy for decision making. They are often an extension of the physician and may influence admitting decisions if the doctor belongs to the admitting staff of more than one hospital. Winning the physician but losing the staff will ultimately lose the physician as well. Successful senior managers will realize this and learn to deal with the staff.

Involve Physicians in Strategic Planning

Senior managers and executives should involve physicians in long-range strategic planning and the administrative decision-making processes. Often, physicians are not accustomed to long-term decision making; most of their day-to-day tasks and decisions are short term. Physicians may become particularly frustrated when policies take many months or even years to implement. They frequently become impatient with what they perceive to be slow and bureaucratic processes. Their advocacy role with patients also makes it difficult for them to tolerate long waits for solutions to problems; often time is running out for their patients.

Deliver What Is Promised

Each promise must be kept. Credibility is established by doing what you say you will do.

Earn Physicians' Personal Respect

Physicians do not respect a senior manager or executive because of the position he or she holds. In fact, many physicians have a strong negative bias against health care administration in general. However, as most physicians get to know senior managers and executives, they come to respect them as individuals. Thus senior executives should develop personal relationships with physicians; they should not rely on the power of their positions to influence the medical staff. Physicians respect doers. Senior managers and executives who are known by the medical staff as people who get things done for them are likely to be effective.

The Physician as a Business Partner

In the past several years, health care organizations have become business partners with physicians for the first time. Although there have been numerous successful ventures, there have also been many failures. Many of the latter are the result of personal failures and have little to do with business issues. The coming years will demand more of such partnerships, and it will become necessary for senior managers and executives to become more personally adept at managing these relationships. The protocols discussed below are useful in the context of the business partnership.

Remember That the Health Care Corporation
Is Dealing with a Smaller Corporation

When senior managers negotiate and ultimately contract with physicians, they are representing a much larger organization than that of the physicians. Their fundamental values are also vastly different from those of the physicians. Physician groups are relatively small and have more private interests. Health care organizations have a great deal of capital backing them as well as imposing resources. Health care executives represent an organization and are not likely to have as much at stake personally in business deals as do the physicians. To the executives, the deal is only one of many organizational issues and concerns. To the physicians, the deal is everything—personally, professionally, and financially.

Remember That Physicians Do Not Move Often

Health care executives should remember that many physicians see administrative staff as people who frequently change employment. A physician's practice, however, is not easily transferred. Because of this difference, doctors do not always believe that health care administrators are as committed to long-range partnerships as they are. Most physicians typically plan to remain in one location for their entire professional life. They have become accustomed to seeing senior health care administrators come and go within their communities.

Physicians Are Not All the Same

The protocols discussed in this chapter are not intended to suggest that all physicians are the same. It can be useful to think of physicians as varying along three distinct lines: stage in their practice life cycle, location of practice, and type of specialty.

Understand the Life Cycle of a Medical Practice

There tend to be profound differences between physicians who have started practicing in the past few years and those who completed their medical training two or three decades ago. Not only is the training different, but the health care system and the methods of reimbursement are dramatically different as well. These differences strongly affect how physicians practice medicine and the relationships they have with health care organizations.

Recent medical school graduates are more likely than older graduates to be female, to come from a wide range of socioeconomic groups, and to have studied medical ethics and business office management. These younger physicians are probably not natives of the community in which they practice and are more geographically mobile. They are also more likely to be willing to work on a salaried basis and are less likely to set up solo practices.

Physicians who have been in practice for a number of years are likely to be more loyal to institutions than are newer physicians. They are likely to have grown up or spent many years in the community in which they practice and thus have strong community ties.

Consider the Physician's Practice Location

Hospital-based physicians tend to be pathologists, radiologists, anesthesiologists, and emergency medicine specialists. Although these individuals may have outside offices, they focus primarily on hospital-based work. As a result, they look to the hospital to provide basic conveniences that doctors who are not hospital-based get through their private offices. Hospital-based physicians seem more attached to the hospital and frequently come in contact with senior health care managers. The protocols that follow are particularly appropriate for these individuals.

Avoid being overly familiar with hospital-based physicians. Health care executives should be cautious not to become overly familiar with hospital-based physicians. Because they see them more often and know them better, senior managers often act more informally and casually with hospital-based doctors than with doctors who maintain outside offices and may also admit to other institutions. Hospital-based physicians may feel taken for granted when compared to outside staff. Thus, it is important to pay close attention to their needs and be certain that resources are shared with areas that are not exclusively targeted at community doctors.

Involve hospital-based physicians in the budget process. Senior managers should make every possible effort to involve hospital-based physicians in the budgeting process for their areas. Because they have little opportunity to meet their needs in outside arenas, they need to know that their needs and wants are given appropriate and sincere consideration during any allocation process. This involvement should be more than an administrative department head carrying the budget decisions back to these physicians. Senior managers should take the time to hear physicians' requests and respond to them on a personal basis.

Consider the Physician's Specialty

In this area the differences are generally very noticeable. Perhaps the sharpest contrast is between surgical specialists and physicians in family practice.

Surgeons are usually involved in comparatively brief interventions. When dealing with them, senior managers should keep in mind that they are action-oriented; they seek to diagnose the cause of problems with expediency and solve them quickly. Surgeons are trained to solve problems with intervention techniques. They tend to be comfortable with technology and to focus on the capital processes within an organization. Family practitioners, in contrast, are people-oriented and comfortable with processes. They focus on issues and are trained to be good listeners.

The following two protocols are helpful in approaching the wide variety of physicians that senior managers will encounter in health care organizations.

Constantly study the differences. Senior managers should always bear in mind the stark differences in physician specialties. They should not approach them all in the same manner administratively. It is helpful to meet with groups of physicians by specialty to more easily learn about and deal with their specialty-specific issues and problems. Answers that might satisfy physicians in one specialty could dissatisfy those in another.

Visit doctors on their home turf. In dealing with community-based specialists who have offices off-site, health care administrators should make it a point to visit them in their offices at least once each year. This will not only build good relationships, it will also build knowledge and awareness of their distinct needs and concerns.

Summary

Protocol is very important to physicians. Of all relationships that have to be appropriately managed, those with these essential members of the health care delivery team are paramount. Because physicians are the preeminent component of the health care organization, the protocols for dealing with them are important parameters of senior management and executive success. It is unnecessary and undesirable for executives to either fear or revere physicians, but it is essential that executives understand them and deal with them appropriately.

Note

1. A. Sheldon, *Managing Doctors* (Homewood, IL: Dow Jones–Irwin, 1986), 86.

Further Reading

Shortell, S. M. *Effective Hospital-Physician Relationships.* Ann Arbor, MI: Health Administration Press, 1991.

12

THE ETHICAL DIMENSIONS OF
HUMAN RESOURCES DECISIONS

Managers are given no greater responsibility than the control and authority they exercise over other people. In every respect, senior managers are guardians of the organization's employees. Employees place enormous trust in their leaders; it is imperative that leaders take this trust seriously and avoid violating it. There is no quicker way to lose credibility and control of an organization than to breach that relationship and allow unethical behavior and decisions in human resources.

Before reading further, it is a good idea to consider—and preferably complete—the human resources ethics questionnaire in Appendix 12.1 at the end of this chapter. Because managers work with people, many of their decisions have ethical dimensions. This questionnaire is designed to assess approaches to different situations by different people.

Ethical Decision Making about Human Resources

Chapter 6 addressed the topic of ethics, focusing on ethics in general, ethics within the workplace and the community, and ethics from a global perspective. There is another element involved in ethical decision making that merits separate attention. It is a dimension of ethics that unfortunately has not received much notice: the decisions that executives make directly affect people.

Although it may sound overly dramatic, senior managers and executives hold the lives of many people in their hands. The human resources decisions they make each day can create enormous burdens for many. The responsibility for other people is one that executives should approach with a great deal of reverence and respect.

The questionnaire in Appendix 12.1 introduced the many issues of human resources ethics. Here are some additional issues with ethical ramifications that executives must address on an almost daily basis:

- Should termination from a position for *inability* to do that job be treated any differently than termination for *insubordination*? Unfortunately, many executives consider only the legal ramifications of these decisions.

- When an employee has a "personality clash" with a supervisor, at what point is it appropriate (ethical) to ask the employee to find another job? This is an all too frequent occurrence, and most organizations almost always side with a supervisor against an employee. The way executives deal with this issue presents ethical challenges for them.

- To what extent is it appropriate for an employer to dictate an employee's outside activities (social, civic, political)? How is it determined whether these activities are having a negative impact upon the organization? As managers move higher up in an organization, the possibility for harm to both the organization and the manager increases. For example, what would be the implications for the organization of promoting a white manager who belongs to an all-white country club?

- How are particular human resources decisions made? What are the guiding principles used in decision making? In one hospital, a competent 21-year veteran secretary was laid off because the wife of the chief executive officer did not like her.

- In another hospital, the pay range for secretaries of vice presidents is three pay ranges higher than that of the departmental secretaries, yet their positions did not factor at that high a level in the hospital's point-factoring job evaluation system.

It is possible to give an endless series of examples of human resources decision making with ethical implications.

Senior managers should consider the ethical implications of the human resources decisions they make daily. They should be certain to address the ethical dimension before making any final decisions or taking action.

The Whole Organization Is Watching

Senior managers should remember that in human resources more than any other area the organization's eyes are on them. Inside the confines of the executive suite, senior managers' unethical actions might go unseen. However, managers' actions that have to do with employees are visible for everyone to see, from the institution's employees to outside legal agencies. Employees watch what happens to their coworkers and have long, detailed memories.

Protocols for Ethical Human Resources Decisions

In any ethical situation, the answer will vary depending upon the circumstances. Decision makers may reach varying conclusions based upon their values, backgrounds, and principles. The needs of and pressures upon the organization will also affect decisions, especially human resources decisions.

Senior managers can incorporate an ethical dimension into their human resources decisions by following the protocols described below.

Consider Guidelines Provided by Religion

These can be excellent guides for behavior. Many health care institutions have religious affiliations, and the organization's denomination may provide a religious context for decision making. The religious tenets of almost every faith address the dignity and worth of the human individual.

Practice the Golden Rule

Many executives have a mental picture of how they hope *they* will be treated if they are terminated. The health care field abounds with stories of senior managers who were dismissed with little or no advance warning and had little to fall back on. Health care executives, whether or not they have had this experience, should approach human resources decision making with compassion and empathy. They should be respectful of the power and authority inherent in their position when making staff decisions. Too often, senior managers and executives remain detached from the effects their decisions have on others.

Practice the Corporate Philosophy

Almost all organizations maintain that people are their greatest resource. Senior mangers should consider to what extent this belief is evident in their human resources decisions.

Know the Laws That Apply to Human Resources

Although following the law does not always mean being ethical, the laws that cover a specific issue often will speak to the correct ethical spirit for the decision. Laws frequently represent the intent of society to be ethical and can provide excellent direction in decision making. Senior managers are urged to consider the spirit and intent of the laws.

Consider Whether Anyone Will Be Hurt by the Decision

This may be one of the most important guiding principles for ethical decision making, particularly in regard to human resources. Obviously, if the decision involves termination (which some call "economic capital punishment"), there is at least one person hurt—the terminated employee. However, some managers may find that an employee who was just terminated actually felt better (or relieved) after being let go.

Consider How Most People Would Feel about This Decision

Many organizations have a rule that states that no employees can be terminated without the approval of either the chief human resources officer, the chief executive officer, or both. This system of checks and balances helps to assure fairness and an ethical approach and gives someone other than the immediate supervisor a chance to review the circumstances and the facts of each case. Ideally, the fairness of termination decisions will improve as a result, and the ethical dimensions will be considered.

Determine the Ideal Situation

Senior managers should always strive to define the perfect model or answer for every human situation. Of course, they will not always be able to achieve the ideal, but thinking about it will help to guide them in the right direction.

Determine Whether Any Good Will Result
from the Decision and Who Will Benefit

This protocol addresses the struggle between the needs of the organization and the needs of the individual. Many decisions involving employees are made because of a supervisor's power or ego and result in no organizational or individual good (except for that supervisor). If no good will result from the decision and no one will benefit, the decision should not stand.

Consider How Best to Maintain a Balance between What Is Good for the Individual and What Is Good for the Institution

This may be the pivotal point on which most ethical human resource decisions are made; almost all such decisions involve this balancing act. Within any organization there is a constant stress (and resulting conflict) between what individuals want and need and what the organization wants and needs. This is further complicated by the fact that the wants and needs of the organization are indeed the wants and needs of more powerful individuals within the organization.

Develop a Rationale for All Personnel Policies

All personnel policies and procedures should have a well-established and well-thought-out rationale. The rationale should be clearly stated with the policy and should set the guidelines under which the policy is enforced.

Establish a System of Due Process for Employees

Senior managers should establish an effective system of due process for employees. This may be one of the most important ethical foundations for any human resources program. A system of due process provides an opportunity for employees to question the decisions of the organization and ensures that justice will prevail as much as possible within the workplace.

Due process at its base level is an organizational system for resolving complaints and conflict. It is more than simply a grievance procedure; it is a corporate attitude that shows that the organization has a sincere interest in its people and their concerns. Managers should not view due process as a win-or-lose situation.

The whole notion of corporate due process is spreading in the United States. It is dealt with in depth in a book by David W. Ewing entitled *Justice on the Job: Resolving Grievances in the Nonunion Workplace.*[1] Ewing reviews the system of due process at several leading U.S. corporations. He notes that these programs emphasize the process, not the answers. The process must have integrity and credibility and employees must be free to use it and must ultimately believe that it can work for them.

Develop a Human Resources Philosophy

Executives should develop a philosophy of human resources. They should determine how they feel about people and how they plan to treat them. This should be done on both a corporate and an individual basis. Most

Exhibit 12.1   A Sample Human Resources Corporate Philosophy
Statement

Saga Corporation: Employee Bill of Rights

Saga employees have:

1. The right to give and receive feedback.

2. The right of fair treatment in every area of work experience.

3. The right to basic dignity, respect, and personal identity as a human being.

4. The right to a style of management that enhances self-esteem and dignity as a person.

5. The right to have the opportunity for a meaningful job for which they are qualified.

6. The right to be consulted and involved in those decisions that relate to their job.

7. The right to be involved in social action programs.

8. The right to set their own work goals.

9. The right to set their own lifestyle.

10. The right to be creative in the performance of the task and in the fulfillment of the daily goals.

11. The right to fair compensation for their efforts.

12. The right to work hard to develop in a way that enables them to meet new challenges.

13. The right to be coached, assisted, and helped in the achievement of their goals.

14. The right to an optimistic, trusting, caring relationship in their work environment.

---

corporations have some type of corporate human resources value statement. The real test is how it is applied. Senior managers are urged to develop a personal set of principles for human resources situations and live by them.

Exhibit 12.1 presents the human resources corporate philosophy statement of the Saga Corporation.

Getting the Organization to Respond to Ethical Issues in Human Resources

The organization that is open and willing to put all of its human resources issues on the table is one that will go far in dealing with the ethical dimensions of human resource decisions. David Ewing talks about this more specifically in *Justice on the Job*. Although his comments pertain to a narrow focus of the working environment, they can conceptually help address wider issues of human resources ethics. One particularly pointed comment by Ewing is the following:

> Ethical conduct cannot always be legislated by management. Sometimes it must be forged in the resolution of conflicts over actual problems. What due process does is allow such questions to be aired and debated in a neutral corner. It succeeds where a code or policy guidebook may fail because it allows situations that cannot be anticipated to become part of the webbing of rules and standards by which employees are bound.[2]

The spirit behind this approach and the corporate willingness to open up and allow controversy to surface are what will make an organization more ethically responsible toward its employees.

Summary

Perhaps the most pressing area for executive protocols is the ethical dimensions of human resources decisions, because such decisions affect people so directly. The entire organization observes and remembers the human resources decisions that managers make. Senior managers who diligently avoid violating the trust given them by the organization's employees will ultimately have loyal and committed employees, which greatly benefits the organization.

Notes

1. D. W. Ewing, *Justice on the Job: Restructuring Grievances in the Nonunion Workplace* (Boston: Harvard Business School Press, 1989).
2. Ibid., 10.

Appendix 12.1: Human Resources Ethics Questionnaire

There are no right or wrong answers. Please answer as you *would* act and not how you think you *should* act. Answer as though you had the complete authority to make the decision. Remember that the question of legality is not at issue in these questions.

1. Effective and efficient screening of applications and résumés matters. Your employment services division makes a quick review of all these applications and résumés and makes certain screening decisions. Some of the applications and résumés are placed into a "dead" file, which means that they will not receive any consideration for any positions. This is an acceptable practice.

Strongly Agree	Agree	Neither Agree Nor Disagree	Disagree	Strongly Disagree

2. It is an acceptable practice to discuss family concerns with candidates for senior positions when relocation and other business-family issues may emerge.

Strongly Agree	Agree	Neither Agree Nor Disagree	Disagree	Strongly Disagree

3. Almost all *external* applicants deserve an explanation of the reason(s) for their rejection when another applicant is selected.

Strongly Agree	Agree	Neither Agree Nor Disagree	Disagree	Strongly Disagree

4. Almost all *internal* applicants deserve an explanation of the reason(s) for their rejection when another applicant is selected.

Strongly Agree	Agree	Neither Agree Nor Disagree	Disagree	Strongly Disagree

5. It is acceptable to designate that certain positions be filled by minority applicants.

Strongly Agree	Agree	Neither Agree Nor Disagree	Disagree	Strongly Disagree

6. Probationary employees who are terminated during the first three months of employment should have virtually *no* appeal rights in the internal organizational grievance procedure.

Strongly Agree	Agree	Neither Agree Nor Disagree	Disagree	Strongly Disagree

7. Certain applicants, such as convicted felons, should never be hired in areas of direct patient care.

Strongly Agree	Agree	Neither Agree Nor Disagree	Disagree	Strongly Disagree

8. Unless prohibited by written contract or statute, an employer should have the right to terminate an employee for any cause.

Strongly Agree	Agree	Neither Agree Nor Disagree	Disagree	Strongly Disagree

9. It is an acceptable practice to use hidden surveillance cameras to detect employee theft when there have been incidents of theft.

Strongly Agree	Agree	Neither Agree Nor Disagree	Disagree	Strongly Disagree

10. It is an acceptable practice to have random locker searches for drugs as long as employees are told beforehand of the possibility.

Strongly Agree	Agree	Neither Agree Nor Disagree	Disagree	Strongly Disagree

11. An otherwise competent managerial employee in the human resources department who becomes an *active* member of a politically extreme group (such as the Ku Klux Klan) should be terminated.

Strongly Agree	Agree	Neither Agree Nor Disagree	Disagree	Strongly Disagree

12. An otherwise competent night shift boiler operator who becomes an *active* member of a politically extreme group (such as the Ku Klux Klan) should be terminated.

| Strongly Agree | Agree | Neither Agree Nor Disagree | Disagree | Strongly Disagree |

13. It is acceptable to make personal phone calls at work.

| Strongly Agree | Agree | Neither Agree Nor Disagree | Disagree | Strongly Disagree |

14. After workers have ten or more years of service with an employer, there is a certain social responsibility to those persons to sustain their employment as long as they are not guilty of serious misconduct on the job. This may mean retraining for new jobs, reassignment to other areas, or creating work for them.

| Strongly Agree | Agree | Neither Agree Nor Disagree | Disagree | Strongly Disagree |

15. When a "personality clash" exists between employees and their supervisors and there are no other jobs to which the persons can easily be transferred, it would be acceptable to terminate the employees before their supervisors.

| Strongly Agree | Agree | Neither Agree Nor Disagree | Disagree | Strongly Disagree |

16. Employees should be allowed to use a formal grievance procedure *only* for specific violations of established hospital policies and procedures (as contrasted with *any* other issues).

| Strongly Agree | Agree | Neither Agree Nor Disagree | Disagree | Strongly Disagree |

17. All employees who steal drugs for any reason should be terminated immediately.

| Strongly Agree | Agree | Neither Agree Nor Disagree | Disagree | Strongly Disagree |

18. There may be situations when human resources managers may discuss with a supervisor information revealed to them in absolute confidence.

| Strongly Agree | Agree | Neither Agree Nor Disagree | Disagree | Strongly Disagree |

19. At work, it is an acceptable practice to distort the truth if it will protect another person.

| Strongly Agree | Agree | Neither Agree Nor Disagree | Disagree | Strongly Disagree |

20. The hiring range for a particular position is $60,000–65,000 per year. A very qualified candidate earning $40,000 per year is the top choice for the position. It is an acceptable practice to hire this person at $50,000 as long as there are no internal equity problems.

| Strongly Agree | Agree | Neither Agree Nor Disagree | Disagree | Strongly Disagree |

21. The degree of support for the annual United Way fund drive or other hospital-sponsored charity may be used as a performance criterion in appraising a *manager's* job performance.

| Strongly Agree | Agree | Neither Agree Nor Disagree | Disagree | Strongly Disagree |

22. It is acceptable practice to take home from work pencils, paper clips, or other small items for personal use.

| Strongly Agree | Agree | Neither Agree Nor Disagree | Disagree | Strongly Disagree |

23. It is acceptable to use the hospital copy machine for making small numbers of personal copies.

| Strongly Agree | Agree | Neither Agree Nor Disagree | Disagree | Strongly Disagree |

24. It is an acceptable practice to take a "mental health day" and call in sick after a busy period at work has ended.

Strongly	Agree	Neither	Disagree	Strongly
Agree		Agree Nor		Disagree
		Disagree		

25. People in general give more to an organization than they receive in return.

Strongly	Agree	Neither	Disagree	Strongly
Agree		Agree Nor		Disagree
		Disagree		

PART III

SERVING THE ORGANIZATION

13

Protocols for Communication:
Oral and Written

Good communication skills are essential for senior managers and executives. It is through communication that all organizational efforts are coordinated and organized. Poor communication is to blame for many organizational problems, and good interpersonal skills are impossible without the ability to effectively communicate. Most of the protocols in this book emphasize good communication skills.

In many respects, communication is the medium whereby competency in all four factors of executive success described in Chapter 1 is demonstrated. It is through effective communications that senior managers demonstrate their proficiency and skills. Communications issues also have a protocol component; there are wrong and right ways to communicate. This chapter describes protocols for communication. It is also suggested, however, that readers supplement these protocols with a good book on communication and its processes.

This chapter addresses oral and written communication. In reviewing the following protocols, remember that oral communication is probably more important. Its impact is immediate; that of written communication is not. The impact of oral communication is immediately observable; that of written communication takes more time. Oral communication reveals the speakers' passion, anger, stress, support, concern, or excitement. Written communication often does not show these as overtly. Oral communication can be personal and intimate and thus often more influential. Written communication can seem impersonal and indifferent.

Oral Communication

Oral communication can be thought of as having two aspects: day-to-day interpersonal communication (including communicating nonverbally and listening), and speech and presentation communication (which is more formalized).

Day-to-Day Communication

Most senior managers are adept in interpersonal communications. Their skill in this area has helped them achieve their present position. However, some subtle areas of communication warrant attention from senior managers.

Provide an opportunity for feedback. Effective one-to-one communication hinges on establishing a dialogue. Both parties should have an equal opportunity for exchange and feedback. Too often though, senior managers and executives do not give others a chance to respond to their verbal messages. Typically they will quickly give instructions or information to others and not wait to ascertain that they are understood. Often this is because of their time constraints and busy schedules. Subordinates can be hesitant to ask for clarification, and all too often the result is misunderstanding.

Even in individual meetings between subordinates and managers the agendas are often so long and the issues so pressing that there is not time enough for a good exchange. Without ample opportunity to receive feedback from subordinate managers, senior managers often become isolated. Many subordinates find the need to prioritize the issues they discuss with their senior managers and streamline and censor the information they provide. Often much information remains unspoken.

Also, senior managers spend a lot of time issuing orders and directives, one-way communications that do not lend themselves to feedback and discussion. Their subordinates understand very well the military model of receiving and carrying out orders. An interesting exercise for senior managers and executives would be to categorize all of their communications with subordinates over several weeks. Most would find that the vast majority of verbal communication falls into the category of directives, orders, or mandates, with little or no time for clarification and feedback.

There are four ways in which senior managers can enhance the give-and-take in situations where they are giving directions and instructions:

1. They should pause frequently to give staff the opening to ask clarifying questions.
2. They should avoid seeming rushed when giving directions.

3. They should ask staff to repeat the instructions to ensure that they understand them.

4. They should go back to the staff later, ostensibly to check on progress but actually to clarify the initial instructions if necessary.

Learn to handle group communications effectively. Executives spend a large amount of time in group meetings where one-to-one communication can rarely take place. Group communication situations lend themselves to competition and gamesmanship. They do not provide a good opportunity for a true exchange. Even within well-developed, closely knit teams, there are always certain types of communications that are too personal and private to be discussed in a group setting. Executives would do well in group settings to (1) keep their messages simple, (2) repeat main points several times, (3) allow plenty of time for questions and answers, and (4) follow up with a written summary of the group meeting. Executives might also want to seek feedback from individuals who were at the meeting to determine the effectiveness of their message.

Take additional time. Because of the need for better one-to-one communication with middle managers, senior executives should set aside ample time for this kind of exchange. They should maintain a regular schedule of individual meetings with their subordinates and should place the emphasis on more time spent in these endeavors rather than trying to streamline the process and minimize one-to-one meetings.

Develop the practice of "Friday issues." Senior managers and executives may find it useful to ask each subordinate to prepare a weekly list of the three or four main issues or problems he or she encountered during the week. Some executives call these "Friday issues" in that they are often prepared on Friday for the executive to review over the weekend. Friday issues need not be formal; a short handwritten summary of the key weekly events will suffice. Establishing "Friday issues" provides informal routine communication that is almost always helpful to senior managers.

Learn to disarm. Senior managers and executives should learn the technique of disarming, in which a speaker brings up during discussion the specific negative points he or she expects others to raise. By being the first to bring up these negative issues, a person can be proactive rather than reactive and defensive. In addition, adversaries lose the element of surprise when the other party is first to raise the problem and immediately proposes points of compromise or solution. Executives should not wait for others to raise their negative issues. If there are no solutions or room for compromises, the executive should state this and the reasons for it early.

Disarming works particularly well in group situations. If it is expected that someone within a group will bring up a tough question or point, leaders may wish to do so first, so as to retain control of the audience. It is especially difficult to look good in front of a group when forced to respond defensively to negative inquiries (particularly if there are no solutions that satisfy the group).

Nonverbal Communication

Senior managers and executives should remember the importance of non-verbal communication. They should manage their nonverbal communication as carefully as they manage their words. Nonverbal communication also includes factors that affect verbal exchange. Office furniture arrangements and environmental factors also send important messages during the communication process. For example, staying behind the desk sends a message of more formality than coming out from behind it to join the other person(s). CEOs who informally drop in on managers to discuss issues send a very different message than they would if they summoned managers to the executive office to discuss the issues.

Dress can also affect communication. For example, keeping a suit jacket on when talking sends a message of formality, whereas taking it off sends a message of informality.

Even where a person sits, particularly in a conference room, can have an impact on communication. Although there can be many psychological aspects of power and influence involved in seating arrangements, sometimes there is no meaning behind the arrangements. Executives need to consider the personality of each group and attempt to determine whether or not there is any significance to seating. One area where seating arrangements can have a psychological impact is in the selection of one's neighbor. One successful nursing executive makes a practice of sitting beside the physician she expects to offer the most conflict in the belief that this arrangement makes it more difficult for the physician to confront and attack her. There is also a certain psychological bonding which occurs during the course of a meeting between people who sit beside each other.

Eye contact and body language. Eye contact, facial expressions, and body language are important nonverbal communication factors.

Eye contact may be the most important, because it reveals interest or distraction, emotion or lack of it, and attention or disregard. Senior managers should attempt to establish and maintain good eye contact to enhance nonverbal communication.

Body language is another important nonverbal communication factor. Much has been written about the signals sent to others by body position. For example, leaning toward a person or keeping the arms unfolded signifies openness. Defensiveness or anger is shown by a more closed body position, such as folding the arms or moving away from a person. The distance that people maintain between themselves is also an important component of nonverbal communication. However, a person's body language cannot always be read accurately. Some people will consciously use their body language to confuse, whereas others will simply contort their body unknowingly. Senior managers and executives should consider what the appropriate physical distance is between themselves and another person. They should not penetrate another's space as this could send an unintended negative or intimate message. Senior managers should also provide nonverbal feedback to speakers, indicating through facial expressions that you heard and understood them.

Listening

Although the emphasis in communication always seems to be on the active area of *presenting*, listening is also important, as was mentioned earlier in this chapter, as well as elsewhere in this book. Executives should listen to determine the effectiveness of their communication, especially verbal communications. Listening can also help determine how to modify or change the content of the message and ascertain how the other person understands it. The following protocols are also helpful.

Remember active listening skills. Executives should use their active listening skills. This requires fighting distractions (such as thinking about the next meeting), listening for the meaning behind what is being said, and looking for areas of personal interest. Executives must avoid "selective listening"— hearing only information that reinforces their point of view.

Pause after communicating. After communicating, senior managers and executives should wait before they make judgments. They should listen for a response from the receiver of the communication. A CEO of an eastern hospital once said, "You must listen to the *person* immediately after you have communicated with them." By this, he meant that it was necessary to hear and understand every response to the message, not just the stated response.

Executives should listen to the verbal message and read the nonverbal message as well and ask for clarification when necessary. They should take extra time to develop opportunities to receive information rather than give it.

Avoid bias and prejudice. Executives should fight against their own biases and prejudices when listening. They should not make illogical mistakes such as mistaking the part for the whole. Consider all messages holistically.

Speeches and Presentations

Senior managers and executives spend many hours in meetings, either hearing or giving presentations or speeches. Presentations and speeches are formal, planned communications. They are very different from day-to-day interpersonal communication, which is spontaneous and candid.

Presentations and speeches generally have higher potential for risk and benefit than informal day-to-day communication. There are several general protocols that can be helpful in making effective speeches and presentations.

Prepare, prepare, prepare. There is nothing more important to an effective speech or presentation than proper preparation. There are two elements of preparation. The first is internal preparation: the speaker's knowledge of the specific material, overall subject area, and the speech or presentation itself. The second is external preparation, including such elements as room location and condition, audiovisuals, and handouts.

There is no better preparation than to thoroughly review the material in a presentation or speech. The best (and often most persuasive) speeches and presentations are made from the heart rather than the mind; this means that the speaker learns the material so well that he or she does not need to refer to any notes or outlines. Speakers who are this well prepared can watch the audience and determine the level of interest and support and the degree to which they are following the speech.

Good speeches and presentations generally sound to the audience like informal conversation. Good persuaders are able to make each person in a group feel as though the communication is targeted at him or her. Speakers who must constantly refer to notes, cards, or outlines will not be able to accomplish this as well.

There is one occasion when the speech or presentation should follow an absolute script: when the content of the speech or presentation must be so exact (usually for legal reasons) that there is no possibility of deviating from specific preselected words and phrases.

Good presenters will often rehearse a speech or presentation. If there are strict time constraints, they will time their delivery. The rehearsals should usually be done before an audience (even of one) to get some feedback on style, content, and delivery.

External preparation relies on others. Any speaker or presenter can be totally prepared as an individual, but he or she may not always be able to control external factors.

Speakers and presenters should have contingency plans for situations such as the following:

- The projector breaks and you cannot show your overheads.
- You bring ten sets of handouts and twenty people show up.
- Your overheads are too small to be read by people in the back of the room.
- You lose your notes for your speech or presentation.
- You are in a room that is much too hot or cold. The meeting room has only one door, located at the front of the room, and you expect people to arrive late or leave early.
- The key decision maker of the group to which you are making a presentation is not in the meeting.
- Your presentation relies very heavily upon a videotape and the tape breaks.

Speakers and presenters should be prepared for all kinds of problems. They may plan to use visual aids, notes, and the like, but they should be ready and able to carry on if something goes wrong.

When the speech or presentation will be given in an unfamiliar room, executives should try to visit ahead of time to get a feel for it and to try out the projector, video player, or other equipment.

Look great and act great. Speakers should never apologize for their presence. A replacement speaker should act as if he or she were the originally scheduled speaker. A speaker with a cold should not apologize for it. Those who feel unprepared should not say so. Any form of apology will allow some members of the audience to immediately tune a speaker out. Furthermore, speakers should not apologize for the room or the equipment or other things over which they have no control. Some of the best presentations and speeches have been made in very poor settings.

Written Communication

There are numerous books that address the basics of written communication. The protocols discussed below present more subtle and intricate aspects of written communication that can affect executive success.

Although verbal communication is more immediate and sometimes much more effective in the short term than written communication, written communication is more significant on a long-term basis because it is longer-lasting and can be studied over time. As a result, written communication is potentially more risky. Memos, letters, and notes have a long life; long after people forget what a person has *said*, they are able to read what a person has *written*. In addition, written communication often is read at a time when the writer is not around to provide explanation or interpretation.

The protocols that follow can help senior managers and executives communicate more effectively in writing.

Develop a Mental Checklist

Before writing, executives should go through a mental checklist. They should identify why they are writing and who will read the message. They should determine if written communication is really necessary. They should decide how the message should be presented—memo, letter, or informal note.

Know When Not to Write

Senior managers and executives should understand when and when not to write. They should *not* write when they are upset or angry; that is the worst time to put thoughts into writing. It is a good idea for a senior manager's secretary to hold for a day or so any correspondence that seems to have been written with anger or strong emotion and the manager look the content over one more time before sending.

Often the timing of a note, memo, or letter is more important than the content. Executives should try to determine the best time to send correspondence.

Written communication should be avoided when face-to-face interaction is called for. If the issue is of a rather personal nature, a face-to-face encounter is usually better than written communication. Even when there seems to be no time for direct personal contact, executives should make the time; it will pay back dividends.

Ideally, senior managers and executives should respond to all written correspondence addressed to them. One hospital CEO made it a policy to answer *every* piece of mail within twenty-four hours. Even though much of that mail asked for information or decisions that would take additional time to research, this executive sent an acknowledgment letter to the sender that indicated an approximate time when the sender could expect further response.

Observe the Ethics of Written Communication

Corporate letterhead is for corporate matters only and the communication that goes out on it should relate to the business of the organization. Executives should use personal stationery and their own supply of stamps for personal correspondence they write at the office.

This protocol is often violated on cover letters sent with résumés by job seekers. This is inappropriate. Even if the job seeker's present employer does not object to this practice, it may raise questions in the minds of recipients about the applicant's sense of propriety.

Send Handwritten Notes When Appropriate

Handwritten notes are appropriate on certain occasions and send a strong personal signal that executives have taken extra time to consider the content of their correspondence. Use handwritten communication to express condolences, personal thanks, or congratulations.

Decide Who Should Receive Copies

Who should receive a copy and who should not is an important consideration. Executives should give careful thought to when and whom to copy. There is no science for determining this; executives must consider each situation on a case-by-case basis. As a general guideline, one's superior should be copied in any situation where it is important to avoid surprising him or her.

Use a Clear Writing Style

Executives should not use jargon or pedantic language. They should write clearly with simple, carefully chosen words and phrases. They should also try to write short sentences and paragraphs. Business writing is not intended for a thesis or textbook. Executives target their writing to the knowledge and level of interest of their recipients.

Clarity can be improved in the following ways:

1. Use concrete, specific phrases rather than vague, abstract ones; and give facts and figures whenever possible. (For example, state "We had a 10 percent nosocomial infection rate" rather than "Our infection rate was really high last year.")

2. Specify action with clear words that readers recognize immediately. (Use "stop" rather than "cease and desist" or "terminate the

employee" rather than "give due consideration and reflection to ending the employment relationship of the employee.")

3. Make specific requests or give specific instructions. (Use: "meet with me no later than next week to conclude our decision on the matter" rather than "let us get together soon to discuss this.")

Develop a Consistent Style

In building an executive image, many senior managers try use a consistent style in their letters and memos. They keep in mind that they are trying to send a message of professionalism and realize that one of the marks of professionalism is consistency.

Executives may want to consider such things as whether to use a middle initial, whether to spell out all abbreviations, and whether to use contractions. All of these small nuances build a consistent style that allows executives to set themselves apart in an acceptable manner.

Use the Same Protocols for Electronic
Mail as for Other Written Communication

The use of electronic mail has been increasing in health care circles, and managers follow the same protocols as for other written communication. Electronic mail sends messages quickly, so executives should avoid sending electronic mail messages during times of stress or strong emotion. Electronic mail is ultimately not confidential and executives should remember that the informality that usually accompanies it can create problems for hasty senders.

Get the Facts Before Writing

When facts are put down in writing, they can easily be tested. Although people may sometimes get by with quoting a wrong number in verbal presentations, they cannot easily do so in writing. Accuracy in written communications is paramount. Inaccurate facts and figures will destroy the credibility of the rest of the message.

Send Notes Expressing Concern or Condolences

Senior managers must communicate frequently in writing when another person has suffered a tragic loss or misfortune (such as a death in the family, a serious accident, or other serious loss). This communication, although very difficult to write, is often appreciated more than any other by the receiver.

By handwriting rather than typing this type of message, executives show that they have devoted extra time and care to the message. Handwritten messages also are more personal. Handwriting must be legible, however.

Usually a short note will suffice in such situations. Executives should state the obvious first—that they are sorry to hear of the loss or other problem and want to express concern to the person. If the loss involves the death of someone the executive is acquainted with, it is appropriate to make some personal comment about the person. A positive observation or reflection might bring some comfort to the receiver of the message. Third, if it is appropriate, executives should offer assistance to the person. This is particularly true if the person was an employee with your organization. Finally, end the note quickly. Do not write on and on.

Summary

Communication counts. Executives should always keep in mind that saying the appropriate thing at the appropriate time, and saying it well, will reflect positively on them. Because communication is the medium by which executives get things done through other people, the importance of communication protocols cannot be overemphasized.

14

PROTOCOLS FOR BUSINESS-RELATED SOCIAL OCCASIONS

"You are cordially invited to a reception . . ."

"We work hard here and we play harder."

"Let me take you to lunch and I will tell you all about this issue."

"We need to get the managers out together for a mixer and help them feel more a part of the team."

"Stop by for our 'attitude adjustment' hour."

"Let's meet for breakfast and cover those issues."

All of the above are characteristic of a key feature of business today, the business-related social occasion. Health care executives are increasingly called upon to appear at a multitude of parties, receptions, lunches, and dinners. To be successful, senior managers must be comfortable at these social gatherings. Business entertaining is an important component of an executive's life.

In health care there are many occasions for entertainment and socializing. Potential business contacts or community supporters may be invited to social functions held by the institution. Many organizations have auxiliaries or foundations that sponsor social events that require executives' participation. The December holidays call for numerous parties and celebrations.

Within the workplace, there are social events that require attendance and participation. The senior managers of an organization often get together socially. The chief executive officer may host these events or the group may have its own customs.

There are a multitude of other circumstances in which executives are faced with situations involving socialization. Many physicians hold parties and receptions both in their homes and in public settings. Community leaders frequently host social gatherings of one kind or the other. There are events in the community that executives are expected to attend as part of keeping up the corporate image, such as fund raisers for social agencies or arts and cultural organizations. These civic events bring health care executives in contact with senior managers from many industries and businesses. Health care executives are expected to mix, mingle, and represent their institutions well.

At many social occasions, people tend to relax too much and forget their manners. Although society condones relaxing and enjoying oneself at social affairs, executives must maintain professional decorum or face the possible consequences.

Social graces are an important part of the fourth factor of executive success. Senior managers and executives should spend some time polishing their social skills.

General Social Protocols

Every executive would do well to read Letitia Baldrige's *Complete Guide to Executive Manners*. In addition, this chapter presents several social protocols for health care executives.

Do Not Overindulge at Cocktail Parties and Receptions

Executives should not attend cocktail parties or receptions just to eat and drink. These social functions are not intended to be all-you-can-eat-and-drink smorgasbords. Although executives should enjoy these events, their primary objective should not be having fun; the purpose of practically all business entertaining is business. A business party is *not* the place to have one's "attitude adjusted." It is an opportunity to meet others, socialize, and mix in a somewhat relaxed atmosphere. Executives should maintain a professional demeanor even in a festive atmosphere.

Senior managers and executives should make it a rule to have only one alcoholic drink at business functions, and they should avoid drinking and driving. They should remember that many other people are watching their behavior.

A corollary to moderation in drinking is moderation at the hors d'oeuvres table. Managers may want to consider eating something beforehand to take the edge off their hunger. They should enjoy what is served but should not eat as though the food is their main interest. Grazing continuously at the food table is uncouth and ill-mannered.

Learn to Mix Easily in Social Situations

Senior managers and executives should be able to mix and talk easily in social settings. They can learn how to do this even if they are not outgoing by nature. Given the business purpose of these events, it is important to make contact with as many people as possible and not stay in one place. When executives "work" a reception or party, they should circle around the room. It is also important to learn how to move from one person to another without seeming rude. Executives should learn the art of social disengagement. Do not stay engrossed in conversations with the same people. Rather, try to introduce new people into the conversation to give yourself the chance to move on to another group.

It is also important for executives to be able to make small talk—about, for example, sports, travel, or current affairs—at these events. They should stay away from controversial issues. A business-related social event is not a proper forum for attempting to win others over to one's point of view. Small talk should be two-way and done with a spirit of sharing. Executives should not dominate the conversations; they should listen to others and learn something about them and their personal interests.

Little Things Mean a Lot

Executives can improve the impression they give by following a few simple guidelines. For example, they should hold their drinks in the left hand so that they do not shake hands with a cold wet hand. Executives should brush up on the guidelines for making proper introductions. This will greatly improve their poise and ease meeting new people.

An executive hosting a gathering should be the first to arrive and should stand at the door greeting guests until everybody arrives. After all the guests have arrived, the host should mix with everyone in the group over the course of the evening. Hosts or hostesses should consider skipping dessert in order to make the rounds at the tables.

Spouses Have a Role

The health care executive's spouse or significant other is an important part the "executive team." This is often considered during interview situations, but it is often forgotten later. Spouses usually are seen only at parties or social situations, although they may do volunteer work in the hospital or participate in the auxiliary.

Because spouses have no organizationally granted authority, they should attend social events as guests and not step into the role of an executive by giving counsel or issuing orders. They should avoid talking about management or issues. Because many spouses have careers of their own, executives should be cautious about making social commitments for them without checking with them.

The Business Lunch

Senior managers often go to business lunches. These may be one-on-one occasions or involve groups of persons. There are several useful protocols for business lunches.

Be a Gracious Host

Executives who are hosting a business lunch should try to make arrangements in advance. In particular, they should make sure the server knows who should receive the check. It is wise for executives to go to restaurants where they know the menu and the service.

The host should be punctual; being on time shows respect for other people and their time. If executives arrive early, they should remember that it is generally considered rude to go to the table first without the guests.

Avoid Drinking at Lunch

It is common courtesy to extend to the guest the opportunity to order an alcoholic drink. However, executive hosts should carefully consider the potential negative ramifications of having even one drink at lunch. A good rule of thumb is to never have any kind of alcoholic beverage during lunch if one plans to return to the office. This avoids creating the perception on the part of others that one has "boozed it up" during lunch. Remember that perception is more important than reality. The polite approach for the executive is to offer the guest the opportunity to order a drink but to quickly add that he or she will not to do so because of a heavy afternoon work schedule.

One western chief executive officer always told the executive team that they should feel free to have a drink at lunch but they should then take the rest of the day off and work at home. This was an *absolute* rule within the organization.

Observe Proper Decorum at the Table

During a business lunch, executives should avoid disputes with restaurant staff. The lunch should be a sidelight to the business agenda.

Respect Others' Time

Early in the lunch, the host should try to find out any time constraints the other parties may have; one person may need to return to the office quickly.

Be prepared to move into the business agenda shortly after the drinks (coffee, tea, alcohol, soft drinks) have arrived. It is inconsiderate to postpone that discussion until late in the meal because there may not be enough time to deal with it.

Do Not Argue over the Check

Never argue over who pays the check. This often presents what is perceived by some as an ethical dilemma. Executives should determine to what extent it is appropriate to allow someone who is in a position to gain something from them to buy lunch.

Although the ethical purist may wish to avoid *all* business lunches so as not to have to grapple with this problem, most executives will encounter such occasions. It is generally acceptable to allow a salesperson, consultant, or other vendor to pick up a lunch check. The appropriate behavior is usually dictated by the type and terms of the business relationship.

Avoid debating over paying the bill. One health care administrator working in an organization with rather strict ethical guidelines created an embarrassing situation with a labor attorney who simply wanted to get acquainted over lunch. This labor attorney took the executive to a private club for lunch where it was impossible for the vice president to pay his share of the bill. Because he felt obligated to obey his strict institutional policy of accepting absolutely no free lunches, he insisted that the attorney take some payment for the lunch. This created great embarrassment for both parties.

The business lunch is also not the time nor place to debate the size of the tip or how the bill may be split when it is shared. Divide it evenly, leave the customary tip, and get on with the business portion of the lunch.

Do Not Smoke

Given the societal trends today, smokers should probably not even ask permission to smoke if their companions do not smoke. Some nonsmokers are not assertive enough to answer that they would prefer that no one smoke.

Summary

Much more could be written about executive behavior at parties and social gatherings, and there are numerous books on the topic. One such book, by Jan Yager, is entitled *Business Protocol: How to Survive and Succeed in Business*. Yager summarizes much of the message of this chapter in the following: "...remember that your behavior, whatever type of entertainment setting is chosen—breakfast, lunch, dinner, party, holiday bash—is always under scrutiny. Good manners and etiquette apply *especially* in these seemingly unofficial settings. Ironically, it may be even more important to scrutinize your every word, as well as what you wear and how much you drink or eat, in these pseudosocial situations, where you might be tempted to let down your guard, than even in the obviously business face-to-face meeting with your boss in his office."[1]

The ability to exhibit grace and good manners at social occasions is an important element of appropriate executive behavior. As managers move higher in any organization, they can expect to attend an increasing number of social events and activities. They should pay cautious attention to their behavior at these events. They should always stay in control and remember that they are at business functions.

Note

1. J. Yager, *Business Protocol: How to Survive and Succeed in Business* (New York: John Wiley & Sons, 1991), 147.

Further Reading

Gelles-Cole, S., ed. *Letitia Baldrige's Complete Guide to Executive Manners*. New York: Rawson Associates, 1985.

15

RECRUITMENT AND SELECTION

When considering appropriate executive behavior in recruitment and selection situations, readers should recall their own experiences both as candidates for positions and as employers interviewing others. They should remember their own interviews at other organizations and consider the positive and negative aspects. It is helpful to think about what elements of their interviews they would change and to think about how they and their organizations conduct searches, especially for senior executive positions.

Some organizations are inconsiderate and use poor techniques when recruiting and selecting employees. Although the major focus of this chapter is on recruiting and selecting senior managers, the protocols apply to all levels.

Readers should consider their own experiences as they work through the quiz given in Exhibit 15.1. It is helpful to keep two situations in mind as they answer "true" or "false": first, the *actual present practice* of their own institution; and second, what they would consider *the ideal practice* to be.

The answers to the questions are less important than the thoughts behind them. The recruitment and selection process is filled with potential for error. Although long-lasting impressions are formed during the process, the people involved often give little thought to the process itself.

Issues in Recruitment and Selection

The abilities to recruit and select staff are important components of executive success. A senior manager's team is critical to getting good results in any organization. Senior managers spend a great deal of time recruiting and selecting staff. As one chief executive officer remarked: "I have been in the field for twenty-four years and I have yet to go through more than six

Exhibit 15.1   Recruitment and Selection Quiz

1. One reason to use a search firm is to avoid talking with rejected candidates.

2. The needs of an organization almost always outweigh the need to be considerate of a candidate's time (for example, it is appropriate to have a candidate who is on-site for an interview wait for however long it takes to deal with an unexpected management issue or to keep candidates waiting to hear whether they have been accepted or rejected for however long it takes for the organization to make its decision).

3. It is appropriate to ask an acquaintance for a confidential reference without asking a candidate's permission, especially when the intent is to simply get a general reading of a candidate.

4. It is appropriate to have candidates arrange their own transportation between airport and institution when traveling for interviews.

5. If candidates do not ask questions pertaining to certain problem areas of an organization, they do not need to be told of them. After all, we do not usually expect job applicants to enter the interview process with information about the internal workings of the organization.

6. It is appropriate to leave discussions of salary and benefits (even discussions of general salary ranges and basic descriptions of benefits) with candidates to the end of the process.

7. All interviewed and rejected candidates deserve some explanation as to the reason for their rejection.

8. It is appropriate to place more emphasis on the positive aspects of an institution and its open position when recruiting candidates than to focus on negative aspects of the job or the organization. After all, much of effective recruiting is sales.

9. A candidate has flown in to your institution for an interview. After you (to whom the person would report) have visited with him or her the night before during dinner, you have determined without any doubt that the person would never work out in the position. As a result, you have eliminated him or her from consideration. You will:

   a. Go ahead and allow him or her to interview the next day because he or she will provide some contrast for other, better candidates.

Continued

Exhibit 15.1 Continued

---

b. Be open and frank and tell him or her that in your judgment the fit is not there and give him or her the chance to fly home early (and perhaps not waste the vacation day).

10. If your institution is providing transportation for a candidate to and from an airport, there is no need to be highly concerned over *who* provides that transportation. In other words, the person picking up the candidate and taking him or her back could be a secretary, a hospital driver, an assistant administrator, or anyone else. (As you answer this, consider also the *kinds* of automobiles in which you have been transported).

---

months when I had an entire management team in place—I have always been recruiting." This person was a very effective health care executive, and the openings had nothing to do with any lack of leadership.

The poor job most organizations do at recruiting is not because they lack the ability to recruit, interview, and select. The process itself is flawed. This discussion is not focused on how to interview or how to attract good candidates, nor is it concerned with the mechanics of establishing selection criteria standards. Instead, it discusses other aspects of recruitment and selection, including the courtesies involved in recruiting and messages sent to candidates, which can affect senior managers and their institutions. Many senior managers and executives have had negative experiences in the interview process, ranging from general impoliteness to large improprieties that have left a permanent negative impressions on the candidates. The following scenarios describe true examples of such negative experiences.

Scenario A

A candidate for a vice president position in a prestigious eastern multihospital organization was picked up at the airport by the chain's administrative fellow and driven to a hotel in an old, dirty car that had dog hairs on the front seat, where the fellow's pet usually sat. The administrative fellow, of course, apologized for this.

Scenario B

A candidate was set up for a day of interviewing with a number of senior managers at a leading southern hospital. The chief operating officer, to whom the candidate would report, was scheduled for a two-hour breakfast meeting. Fifteen minutes into their meeting, the chief operating officer was paged and had to call the hospital. By the time he had finished with the crisis, he only had thirty minutes with the candidate. There was no opportunity later in the day to make up the time. Several weeks later the candidate was told by the search firm consultant that another candidate had been selected. The rejected candidate was convinced that a lack of time with the chief operating officer was a key factor in not being selected for a follow-up interview.

Scenario C

An eastern hospital, working through a search firm to recruit a corporate vice president for its three hospitals, brought in the top three candidates recommended by the search consultant. A finalist was brought back for a second two-day visit and was then invited back with his spouse for a third visit. During this visit, the candidate and his wife spent two additional days touring the area with a realtor and another day meeting hospital staff.

After this final visit, three weeks passed without a formal offer. The candidate finally received a call from the search firm consultant. The organization had asked the consultant to start the search again from scratch. There had been an internal struggle between the system president and the administrator of the flagship hospital over the appropriate type of candidate for the position. The leading candidate, although he met the requirements of the chief executive officer perfectly, did not meet the criteria of the administrator of the flagship hospital. The search was started over again, and a totally different type of candidate was presented.

It is tempting to dismiss this scenario as just an unfortunate circumstance for the rejected candidate who spent so much time interviewing; such rejections are an unfortunate but common part of executive life. However, the health care industry is small and this kind of organizational behavior, which is counter to the caring philosophies most often expressed by health care organizations, should be avoided. The organization should have worked out the exact specifications for the position before wasting the candidate's time.

Scenario D

A competent senior health care vice president was interviewing at a local hospital for a lateral position. Her hospital's chief executive officer had recently left, and she believed that it would be a good time to pursue another opportunity. This one was particularly attractive because it was local and the hospital had a national reputation.

The initial interview with the chief operating officer took place during the second week of January and went quite well. The candidate was advised that she would definitely be included in the second round of interviews. During this early interview, a rather specific salary discussion increased the candidate's expectations.

During the third week of February, the candidate called the chief operating officer to check on the progress of the search. The chief operating officer expressed continued strong interest in the candidate and indicated that he would get back to her in a few days.

The candidate received a call from the chief operating officer's secretary during the second week of March to set up interviews with seven individuals, including the hospital's chief executive officer, on six different days over a total period of fifteen days. The candidate agreed to all the interviews. At this point, the confidentiality of her candidacy was severely compromised because she had to risk being seen so many times.

During each visit to the hospital, which had no central executive suite, the candidate was left on her own to find each office. For six of the seven interviews, the candidate was kept waiting at least ten minutes past the appointed time for the interview. One appointment even began forty minutes late.

During the first week of April, the candidate received a call from the chief operating officer informing her that she was one of two finalists and would be scheduled for an interview with the hospital's consulting psychologist. Three weeks later the candidate was asked by the psychologist's secretary to meet in the psychologist's room at a local hotel. When the candidate asked for another date that would better fit her calendar, she was told that she would have to see the psychologist then because he did not have another time slot available for three weeks and the hospital was anxious to finish the selection process that week.

The psychologist's tests and the interview itself seemingly had little or no relation to the position. Three weeks after the candidate had met with the psychologist, the chief operating officer called to express his regrets that the institution had decided to employ another individual. When asked for the reason, the candidate was told that it was "chemistry," rather than anything specifically lacking in her experience. When she asked who had been selected, she was told that information could not be released yet because negotiations were still ongoing.

Later the rejected candidate learned that the hospital had hired an individual with no hospital experience. It seems that the chief executive officer had preempted the chief operating officer's decision. The candidate felt that her time with the chief executive officer had been rushed and that had been a contributing factor in the selection.

Scenario E

In the same city where Scenario D took place, another chief executive officer recruited a number of senior managers for her staff. Several rejected candidates commented on the process. Even the rejected candidates had a positive opinion of the hospital and the chief executive officer. This executive spent a great deal of time with the candidates she rejected, trying to help them understand the process and why they had not been chosen. She believed that an organization should show as much sensitivity as possible when recruiting senior executives.

These examples illustrate how ordinary recruitment can be mishandled and thus create very negative perceptions of the organization. On the other hand, when it is managed well, recruitment can create a positive impression of the organization.

Protocols for Recruitment and Selection

If senior managers and their organizations follow the protocols discussed below, they will enhance their reputation for being caring and sensitive recruiters and maximize their chances of hiring their first-choice candidate.

Become Known as an Organization with
Impeccable Recruitment Technique

Senior managers and executives can distinguish themselves and their organizations from others by how well they handle the interview and selection process. In the long run, those who spend extra time and effort can achieve more productive interviewing, attain a greater reputation, and ultimately gather a stronger team.

Set Standards for the Interview Process
and Treat All Applicants Equally

Most institutions allow daily activities to interrupt the interview process. Many institutions treat the entire interview process haphazardly. Most senior managers have had an unpleasant interview experience, including, for example, last-minute schedule changes, interviews starting or ending late, and lengthy waits outside different executive offices. Interviews cannot always be perfectly orchestrated; in health care, issues arise that must be handled immediately. However, senior managers should consider the recruitment process from the candidate's point of view and make every effort to keep disruptions to a minimum.

Design the Interview So That the *Experience* Is Consistent and Structured

A structured interview process eliminates the haphazard nature that interviews often have and helps to ensure that minor courtesies and protocols are not overlooked or forgotten. Behavioral experts maintain that this approach will make the process more objective and increase the likelihood of a more informed decision. In addition, doing so will improve an institution's reputation for having a high-quality selection process. This will be important in the coming years; as the predicted labor shortages affect health care organizations and allied health personnel become scarcer, institutions that treat applicants as *customers* will be most effective at recruiting the most desirable candidates.

Interview Others as You Would Like to Be Interviewed

Although this protocol is simple, many organizations do not practice it. For example, a senior manager should meet the candidate at the airport (this basic courtsey is seldom practiced). Senior managers should be certain that candidates receive ample information about the location (real estate information as well as community information), the organization, and the job for which they are interviewing (unfortunately many candidates are sent rather paltry information).

Senior managers should make sure that the hotel knows that the candidates are VIP guests and bills the room and meals directly to the hospital. Managers should inspect the kinds of rooms candidates will occupy and speak with the hotel manager to ensure that the staff pays particular attention to the candidates' needs.

If a candidate is invited for a second visit, send some sort of welcoming gift, such as a fruit basket or flowers, to the candidate's room. Recruiting is in many respects a courting process in which managers and their organizations woo the candidate from another organization.

During a long day of interviews, consider the candidate's personal needs. It is interesting how many organizations will shuttle a candidate from interview to interview without a break.

Managers should start and end interviews on time and be sure that candidates do not waste time waiting to see the next interviewer. When there are unavoidable interruptions, they should try to provide the candidates with some appropriate reading material.

Respect and Honor Confidentiality

All too often senior managers act as though candidates have given up their rights to confidentiality. Most good candidates do not want their present employers to know of their interest in another position. Managers should make a special effort to protect every candidate's confidentiality.

However, it is easy to violate a candidate's confidentiality. For example, an executive on the interview team who knows another executive in the same town might make a confidential call and ask about the candidate. Even worse, an executive in the interviewing organization might call a schoolmate or other close colleague working in the *same* organization as the candidate. Or an executive might call someone who recently worked in the same organization or a physician might call a colleague at the organization.

Such breaches of confidentiality occur quite frequently. In health care, many executives have large networks. Some people believe that there is no problem with making inquiries such as those described above; that this is the risk that candidates run when they interview for new positions. Such an attitude is most unfortunate. In reality, any conscious breach of confidentiality is wrong unless the candidate gives permission. Once senior managers begin to officially check references, they should make certain that candidates understand that they may check more than just those listed by the candidate.

Offer the Candidate a Realistic Job Preview

Senior managers should provide all applicants with an honest and upfront view of the job and the organization. The use of a realistic job preview is based on sound research that has shown that applicants should be given as comprehensive a look at a job and company as possible. Research has shown that candidates who are given a *complete* positive and negative job preview (1) are more likely to self-select out from consideration if the position is unsuitable; (2) have a more reasonable and realistic set of expectations about a job when they begin work; and (3) are less likely to be disappointed, angry, or dissatisfied.

Health care is known for using a hard sales pitch when recruiting and interviewing and for emphasizing the positive aspects of a position and an organization while ignoring the negatives. This is especially true when the hospital is recruiting for scarce staff positions, such as registered nurses and physical therapists. Following the principles of realistic job preview means that an organization does not sell a job or an institution that does not quite exist. It means being as ethical as possible in describing the issues facing the candidate who takes the position.

The following are tactics an organization might use to oversell itself or a position:

- A vice president candidate is promised additional staffing support, although this is never precisely spelled out in a prehire contract.

- An executive is urged to take a position without having had the proper amount of time to really get to know a community and its schools.

- The organization pressures the candidates in the last few days of interviewing. Once the finalist is given an offer, the institution pushes hard for a quick response. Often institutions seem to feel that they can take as much time as they need to select the finalist but then place a strict time constraint on the candidate for a decision.

- Many organizations prefer to wait until very late in the interview process before getting down to the details of benefits and salary. Although they may say they want to get the best candidate first and consider the cost second, in reality they may take advantage of candidates by encouraging them through the process when they know they cannot meet the candidates' salary requirements. Some candidates would not return for second or third visits if they knew the salary and benefits.

Handling Internal Candidates

In the health care industry, there tends to be little opportunity for internal promotion; other industries have a much better track record of promoting from within. Although a number of health care institutions claim to have sophisticated succession planning programs, the overall industry record is weak. Most managers find that they must leave their organizations to advance their careers.

Senior managers must use great caution when the selection process includes internal candidates. Many of these internal candidates have ability and valuable inside knowledge. Sometimes the desire to seek talent with new ideas from the outside is overrated. A strong policy of promotion from within whenever possible will build a solid and loyal management team.

The following are some general protocols for dealing with internal candidates.

Respond on a Timely Basis to Internal Candidates

Carefully plan your response to internal candidates. Institutions typically communicate very little to the internal candidate and often let a long time pass without updating him or her on the status of the search. Internal candidates for senior positions sometimes receive their first notification that they are not being considered for a position when they hear about the person who has been hired.

If internal candidates are not viable, let them know at the beginning of the process. There is nothing more unethical and inhumane than to allow persons to linger for months on the hope and promise of receiving a promotion.

Do Not Give Courtesy Interviews

If internal candidates are not viable, do not put them through courtesy interviews. The particular target here is the traditional health care custom whereby eight to ten people interview a candidate in a day-long marathon. There are other ways to address the concerns of those who say that internal candidates should have the opportunity to practice interviewing or those who wish to prove to the internal candidates that they are indeed not qualified. The interview process itself should be *sincere* and candid.

Do Not Use the Internal Candidate as a Shill

Sometimes, internal candidates are cycled through an interview process only to make external candidates look stronger. There is, in reality, little chance they will be selected. Internal candidates have an uncanny ability to see through the process and invariably understand that they are being used for negative contrast.

Treat Internal and External Candidates Alike

When internal candidates come for their interviews, managers should *interview* them and not discuss organizational business. They should resist the temptation to conduct even a small amount of business or to deal with extraneous issues.

Act Quickly When Dealing with Interim Managers

If the internal candidates are the acting or interim managers in the spot for which they are interviewing, senior managers should speed the hiring process along. A number of health care institutions keep interim managers for more than a year and then bring in an external hire that that person is expected to orient and train.

The Executive Search: From Both Sides of the Desk

The health care industry has seen an explosive growth in the use of executive search firms. There are few senior managers or executives in health care who have not talked with a search firm or consultant about a position. For some reason, however, there appears to be a mystery about what search firm consultants do. There are also some great variations in their practices.

In this chapter, the first set of protocols for using search firms applies to employers who are using the firm to find a candidate. The second set applies to candidates who work with a search firm to find a new position. However, it is useful first to outline the main types of search arrangements and to point out some of the key reasons to use a search firm.

Types of Search Arrangements

There are two primary types of search agreements. The first is the exclusive arrangement or retained search. In this arrangement, the employer typically agrees to work with one firm exclusively and engages its services to find suitable candidates. The employer usually does not do any advertising or recruiting. The search firm receives a set fee (plus expenses) for handling all of the identification of candidates for the client employer. Even if the employer finds a suitable candidate through other means and hires that person, the fee is still owed to the exclusive search firm.

The other popular arrangement is called a contingency search. In this arrangement, an employer hires a firm to identify one or more candidates and pays the firm *only* if one of those candidates is hired. The employing organization is free to use multiple contingency firms and also is able to recruit through its own means. If the organization finds its own candidate, it pays no fees.

Some search consultants, usually the exclusive retained-fee firms, will insist that the retained firm works on behalf of the employer client, whereas the contingency firms work more on behalf of the people seeking positions. A number of contingency firms have generated negative publicity and bad reputations because they made improperly screened referrals. Exclusive firms almost always spend a great deal of time interviewing candidates and check-ing references, whereas many contingency firms simply forward résumés. Exclusive firms also typically have consultants who have worked within the health care industry and have in-depth knowledge of the field.

There are an increasing number of health care search firms competing for lucrative fees. Because exclusive firms also receive reimbursement for expenses incurred in the identification and interviewing of candidates, their financial risk is minimal. A number of employers incur large expenses for candidate identification without full awareness at the outset of the potential for that expense.

In a third type of search arrangement, a firm is hired on a fee-for-service basis to handle specific functions, such as screening candidates or checking references. In this arrangement, the firm bills only for services provided to the employer, whether or not a candidate is found by them.

Protocols for Employees Who Are Using a Search Firm

Although most of these protocols are for organizations using exclusive retained search firms, many of them also apply to contingency firms. A search firm can often be quite helpful to an employer. Exhibit 15.2 details the reasons a health care organization should consider using a search firm. Once an organization decides to engage a firm, the simple protocols described below will help ensure a successful result.

Communicate thoroughly before the search begins. Extensive communication should take place before the search consultant begins so that each party knows exactly what is expected and what to communicate to candidates. In search relationships, the potential for communication problems is huge. For example, an organization may want to hire an executive in the $85,000–$90,000 range. The consultant is advised that $95,000–$100,000 is not totally out of the question, but it is only for the right candidate. The consultant believes that permission was granted to discuss a starting salary of up to $100,000 and communicates it to several candidates. Of course, those candidates have inflated salary expectations. In reality, the employer would have preferred to hold this higher salary out until the last serious negotiations with a finalist. The organization hoped to use the $100,000 amount to seal a deal or to lure an extremely strong candidate who met *every* criteria.

Unfortunately, many executives believe that they can simply ask the search firm to go out and find someone. This leads to confusion later in the process.

Keep in mind that the search firm represents the employer. Senior managers should discuss in advance how they expect all candidates to be treated and handled. If the search consultant is handling too many searches, candidates might not receive the best treatment. Managers should also make certain that

Exhibit 15.2   Reasons for Using a Search Firm

1. A search firm consultant can provide some traditional management consulting. The consultant can give counsel on an organization's needs and inform senior managers of what other similar organizations are doing. The consultant can help define the position or give advice on how to approach problems or system issues.

2. Search firms can help identify market salary ranges and peculiar aspects of a search that may not be immediately apparent to the employer.

3. Many employers do not have the time or the expertise to handle certain kinds of searches. The search firm can provide this needed expertise.

4. Sometimes organizations need to begin searches confidentially so as to have a candidate identified prior to the departure of the incumbent manager.

5. Many senior managers and executives will not respond to (or are not aware of) newspaper or journal advertisements. They will more often respond to a search consultant's call.

6. A search firm can cast a wider net for the identification of candidates.

7. Often a search firm is helpful in bringing objectivity to the process. This is often true when there are internal candidates.

---

the firm gives complete service for the retained fee. Clarify exactly what is expected up front.

Discuss in advance a budget for search expenses. This will avoid unpleasant surprises later. Also, good search consultants handle more than one search assignment at a time and can save money for all their clients by combining expenses. Insist on itemized expense statements. Many firms will simply place a number on their invoice for expenses and add it to the retainer amount. Insisting that the firm presents itemized expenses makes it more careful in its billing.

Spend time with the search consultant during the search process. Plan a set schedule for routine progress conversations. Anticipate problems to arise along the way.

Involve the firm in final salary negotiations. The search firm can serve as a helpful intermediary in the negotiation process. Both parties often are more open with the search consultant than with each other. If the firm is involved in these negotiations, managers should be certain that the parameters are well defined.

Protocols for Job Candidates Who Are Contacted by a Search Firm

Senior managers who are contacted by a search firm to be a candidate for a position should follow the protocols described below.

Determine how much time to spend talking with search firms. A call from a search firm may help one's ego or whet one's curiosity, but such calls also can consume a great deal of time. The time spent on these calls can be quite worthwhile, however. Managers can gain a great deal of information, and the calls may describe wonderful opportunities. Frequent calls, however, may require a considerable time commitment.

Make referrals to the search consultant. Managers should always take the time to talk to search consultants. This is an excellent way to network and to get ideas about what is occurring nationally. Executives should help consultants by referring them to qualified prospects.

Be prepared for search calls. Most senior managers are potentially in the job market and should be prepared for calls from search consultants. Keep an *American Hospital Association Guide* close at hand to get some initial information during the first conversation. Many consultants try to keep the identity of their client confidential until they determine an executive's interest and qualifications. If they are unwilling to reveal the institution, executives can use their own resources to determine it. It is a good idea to keep an atlas nearby to determine geographic location. Association directories have valuable information on the background of the senior executives at the institution described.

Remember the consultant is screening while he or she talks. Unless an executive is known to the search consultant, the initial phone call is a screening interview. Executives should be prepared for this and have at hand a logical and progressive outline of education, work experience, and accomplishments.

Take notes. During the conversation, executives should write down as much detail as possible on the descriptions given by the search consultant. Some senior managers also keep a list of pertinent questions to ask search consultants. They consider these questions important for helping them to determine their own level of interest in the position.

Do not hesitate to inquire about the planned starting salary of the position. Executives should be sure to ask this up front on the phone, before time is wasted meeting the search consultant at the airport or elsewhere. Be as assertive as possible in getting salary or other pertinent information. The majority of firms clarify this in detail with the employer before starting a search assignment. Executives can waste time or risk professional exposure with a potential employer whose salary offer or other benefits are far below their expectations.

Keep an updated résumé at all times. All senior managers and executives should keep a supply of résumés ready for quick mailing. They also should have their résumés reviewed by other executives who make hiring decisions and search consultants accustomed to working in health care.

Mailing a résumé is a personal expense. Cover letters should be on personal, not business, stationery. Executives should type the letter themselves or have it done by a typing service, a family member or friend, or a trusted employee on off-time.

Ethical issues. All of these guidelines and rules may be exempted in the event of an outplacement situation. Many senior managers do not follow these guidelines at all. However, working with executive search firms involves implicit ethical dilemmas, and it is important to be as clear as possible in your own mind about where you stand with regard to the nature of your interaction with these firms and how much you disclose to your own organization. Senior managers who are not clear about their own position may have difficulty avoiding problem areas and unethical temptations. Define your position and stick with it.

Handle meetings with search consultants professionally. Executives who meet with a search consultant should observe the following basic rules:

- Arrive on time
- Bring an additional copy of your résumé
- Bring an organizational chart showing your position
- Be prepared to demonstrate specific measurable accomplishments in your positions
- Allow ample time for the interview

- Be prepared to discuss salary and relocation needs
- Be prepared to express interest (or no interest) at that time or very soon after the interview

Senior managers and executives should not assume that these suggestions are too basic. Search consultants often find candidates unprepared for these meetings.

Interview Protocols for Job Candidates

The following protocols are not intended to provide comprehensive coverage on interviewing; there are a number of good books on this topic. The intent here is to mention a number of key protocols that should be kept in mind when interviewing.

Arrive early and tour the institution. If possible, executive candidates should arrive the day before the interview and take a walking tour of the institution. Talk with the staff and get a feel for the organization.

Get additional information and compare it with that given by the search consultant. Attempt to rectify any concerns or conflicts early in the process. Typically, the longer discussions go along between two parties the less likely they are to retract their positions. One candidate expressed concern with the reporting relationship for the position early in the interview process. The relationship was changed by the chief executive officer at the time, and an agreement was eventually made. It is highly unlikely that the change would have been made had this concern not been mentioned until much later in the process.

Prepare for sensory overload. Overload often occurs if the candidate sees nine or ten people during the day. Remember that a candidate's enthusiasm, energy, and sales ability must be as sharp during the last interview as during the first.

Practice interview skills. Although not all senior managers are in the job market, it might be wise for them to occasionally (every two years or so) test the market. Not only does this provide good interviewing practice, but it can also provide professional stimulation and help refocus goals and accomplishments.

Learn to listen and speak. Executive candidates should work hard to develop the key interviewing skill of maintaining a balance between listening and speaking. For the candidate, this balance is a most difficult one. Without the proper amount of listening, it is hard to learn much about the position, the organization, and the person to whom the interviewee would report. On the other hand, if the candidate listens too much and does not speak enough, the organization may not stay interested in him or her.

Be courteous to everyone. Executive candidates should be particularly courteous to administrative secretaries, other support staff, and administrative residents and fellows. Many chief executive officers use them to transport or escort senior-level candidates around the organization during the interview process and later ask them for their opinion of the candidates.

Summary

The importance of recruitment and selection cannot be overemphasized. The dynamics of change are more frequently caused by turnover and vacancies within organizations than by any other factor. As new people come to an organization and former people leave, the culture within that organization undergoes a great deal of stress. Senior managers who pay attention to the selection process enhance their ability to respond positively to this stress.

Although the major focus in this chapter has been on recruitment and selection at senior levels, many of the protocols and the meaning behind them can and should be applied at all levels. As competition within the industry further increases, the senior managers and executives who excel in these areas will have an edge over the competition.

16

TAKING CHARGE:
STARTING A NEW POSITION

There may be no more important time for senior managers and executives than when they first take over a new position. This period often sets the tone for the duration of their time in the position. The consequences of starting off on the "wrong foot" can be devastating.

There is frequent turnover in the health care industry; in an unpublished study of health care administrators, alumni of The Ohio State University's graduate program in hospital and health services administration, indicated that a majority expected to have to (and would) leave their present health care employers to further their careers. The American College of Healthcare Executives, the American Hospital Association, and the search firm Heidrick and Struggles conducted a study that indicated high turnover among hospital CEOs in the 1980s.[1] Although turnover may have decreased some since that study, readers probably know many acquaintances and colleagues who have moved into new positions and organizations during their careers.

Because senior managers frequently move to new organizations, they should consider protocols for beginning their employment in a new setting. A senior manager's early days and months at a new position in a new organization are crucial to future success. Managers should strive to set the appropriate tone and send the correct signals.

During this initial period, a new senior manager's behaviors are closely watched. Just as society observes the first hundred days of a U.S. president's term in office, organizations closely examine everything new senior managers do and say.

Using Symbolic Behavior

The use of symbolic behavior is particularly important when an executive first takes over a new position. A symbolic behavior can be an action, an inaction, the choice of a word, a gesture, a body movement, or even the choice of a certain suit of clothes. Each of these represents something to others and may send powerful intended or unintended messages. The following protocols will help managers in a new position to begin on the "right foot."

Give a Positive First Impression

In the first days on a new job, senior managers and executives should pay special attention to dress, deportment, hygiene, and other aspects of personal image. During the first few days on the job, new executives should wear "interview clothes" and to be sure that they are immaculately groomed.

Be on Time

Executives during a "taking-charge" period should be on time; any tardiness sends the wrong message to superiors and to subordinates. To subordinates, it can send the message that the new manager feels superior to them; to superiors, such as board members or more senior executives, it sends the message that the new manager does not value their time.

Communicate Clearly

A new manager's first written and verbal messages will be carefully examined by the organization, and especially by subordinate managers. New executives should carefully select their words in these communications and be certain that they say what they mean and mean what they say. This is not a time to be ambiguous or vague. During these first meetings and other communication opportunities, new managers' messages must explicitly communicate their ideas and meanings.

A new chief executive officer at a western hospital sat in the back and observed at his first middle-management meeting; he did not take charge of the meeting. When the group's chair asked at the end of the meeting whether he wished to make any comments, the new chief executive made only a few poorly thought-out remarks from the rear of the room. Most of the middle managers interpreted that to mean that he had little regard for them, their business, and meetings in general. They were disappointed that he had not revealed more of his thoughts and plans. This performance harmed his potential for success within that organization.

Display a Strong Work Ethic

During the first few weeks in a new position, senior managers should send the signal that this is the *most important* opportunity in their career. Spending extra time at the office is one way to send this message.

There is an interesting debate about whether it is more valuable to arrive early or stay late. There are those who say that coming to work early states to the work force and the boss that one cannot wait to get started. This may be an important signal to send in the first few months of one's employment. Staying late, some believe, sends the message that the executive has not been efficient during the day and must stay late. Obviously, there is no right or wrong answer. The amount of time a new executive spends on the job during the first several months makes a strong and lasting statement about his or her degree of interest and loyalty. He or she may also need additional time to learn the organization's history, policies, and other nuances. Whether or not it seems a large part of a new position, the quantity of time spent on the job during the first few months ranks high in people's perceptions of organizational results.

Articulate a Personal Philosophy

New managers and executives should prepare some "philosophical statements" that communicate succinctly their management principles. These should consist of memorable themes and short phrases, and they should articulate these frequently in the first several weeks in a new position. Such interaction will help employees get to know the new manager and his or her managerial style and value system.

One very successful chief executive officer spent the first several weeks at each new job meeting with various groups and summarizing her expectations in six key phrases—teamwork, risk taking, bureaucracy busting, accountability, heroes and outlaws, and initiative. Although the definitions and explanations of these are not important for this discussion, the method is. These phrases provided a "platform" through which she could describe herself, her expectations, and the direction she planned for the organization.

It may be helpful for new managers to view the first few weeks on a new job as the start of a political campaign. A new politician entering a campaign develops a few key issues he or she believes to be important to the constituency and sums up these issues with slogans. The slogans get the attention of those who might not pay attention to an entire speech. Starting a new position involves more than just using political sound bites. The theory behind this approach and its methods are quite helpful for those who must meet with many organizational constituencies. Using sound bites is a simple way for a manager to convey beliefs, directions, and cultural issues to these constituencies.

Be Consistent

Senior managers should establish their credibility by being consistent in moods, work habits, and interpersonal relationships. Consistent behavior makes people comfortable with the new person in power.

Spell Out Expectations

Managers taking over a new position should go to great lengths to spell out what they expect from their subordinates. They should carefully explain the rationale behind their work plans and directions. In essence, during this period senior managers must become excellent teachers and clearly articulate what is behind their ideas and actions.

Take Control Now

Senior managers in a new position should discover how and why the organization does things. They need to possess an auditor's curiosity when learning about organizational approval levels and systems. To adequately do this, managers should question all activities that flow through or around their areas of responsibility. Although many people in the organization will not appreciate this, it often is necessary if new managers are to fully understand what is going on in the organization.

Listen, Listen, Listen

Newly appointed managers should learn as much as possible about the organization. Most people are very anxious to show a new manager what they know and will often tell a great deal more if the new senior manager appears to be a willing listener.

Deliberate, but Do Not Procrastinate

During a new manager's "honeymoon" period, it often is possible to postpone some decision making; it is not expected that new senior managers will have all the necessary facts for making certain decisions. However, soon decisions must be made; the new manager must avoid confusing deliberation with procrastination.

Deliver on Promises

Following through on promises made during the first several weeks in a new position is an excellent way to develop credibility rapidly. Everyone will remember what was promised and accomplished. The credibility of the new senior manager is probably on trial more during this initial period than at any other time. Executives should keep a written record of any commitments they make and check it against their accomplishments on a regular basis. Failing to follow through on promises can cause a permanent loss of credibility.

Use the "1–1–3–7 Guide"

Senior managers and executives might try to divide their first few months on a new job into four segments. After the first week on the job (the "1" of the guide), senior managers should prepare a written list of the five key problems they have identified and the five key movers and shakers with whom they will have to work to succeed. They should keep this written guide for their personal use only and should update it every few weeks. This will provide a written record for testing reality and their ability to read the organizational horizon.

After the first month (the second "1" in the guide), managers should prepare a written list of five to eight expectations that detail what is expected for the first six months in the new position and a list of five to eight very visible changes that could be made easily and quickly.

These expectations should be in the form of generic statements of behavior that can be easily verbalized to any group in the organization. This will help managers to begin to understand what is expected of them and what the key themes and values behind organizational change will be. During this period, senior managers should exhibit a lot of their core values and describe behaviors that they expect to emanate from these values.

One successful health care executive used phrases such as "organizational integrity," "doing the right things the first time," "serving others," and "being effective risk takers." This executive then utilized these key phrases in as many meetings as possible and in private one-on-one meetings with other managers.

Having five to eight ideas for changes that can readily be accomplished provides a logical and effective means of gaining a foothold in the bureaucracy and developing a reputation as an executive of action. After the third month on the job (the "3" in the guide) managers should prepare a written summation of the key problems or issues and present it to the management of the organization (or to the divisional management team). If this is done too early in the new manager's tenure, he or she may have missed some of the more covert problems and the list of problem issues will be roughly the same as a list of problems identified during the interview process. Also, by the end of the third month, senior managers and executives should have had the opportunity to meet personally with all of the key managers within the organization.

After the seventh month (the "7" of the guide), new managers should formally articulate a specific short-term plan of action to take the organization through its first pivotal time period with the new senior manager.

The time frames for the 1–1–3–7 guide may differ slightly for different senior managers. Certain key issues such as a union organizational drive, a serious budget cycle, or impending employee reductions may speed the timetable up substantially. How the previous senior manager or executive left may also affect the plan. This approach is less an effort to codify a specific time frame than an attempt to provide a guideline for action.

It is strongly advised that all new senior managers and executives develop a plan of action with specific deadlines and parameters for guiding behavior in the "taking-charge" phase of a new job.

Display Strengths

During the first few months on the job, new managers should make certain that their strengths are as visible as possible. If finances are a forte, they should spend time and effort on financial feasibility studies or other similar issues. If an executive excels at developing interpersonal relationships, he or she should spend time out of the office doing what comes naturally and pays the largest rewards. If working with physicians is a strength, an executive should focus time and effort on the medical staff. Conversely, this is the time that managers should keep weaknesses as invisible as possible.

Be Cautious

The first few weeks on the job are the wrong time to show impatience or other negative personality traits. During this honeymoon senior managers should be cautious and get to know the organization and people. They should consider what other senior managers and executives have done in other organizations when they took charge and apply the best techniques.

Build Interpersonal Influence

New managers should observe what gives certain people interpersonal influence within the organization and which leaders, both formal and informal, are crucial to a successful transition. New managers should try to get these people to become a nucleus of support for the new policies, practices, and directions.

One new CEO achieved this by simply asking each subordinate manager in the organization to name its one or two most influential people. This list gave the executive a good sense of what the organization valued in interpersonal leadership style. A side benefit was that he also knew to whom he should turn for help.

In every organization a new person must deal with the expectations of others. The process of exploring mutual expectations is vital during the initial few months of the job. A list of changes that could be easily made should include a number of the wishes others articulate during the orientation process.

Senior managers and executives should work as speedily as possible to assemble their own management team. They should assess the existing managers quickly, decide who stays and who goes, hire any replacements, and state their expectations for the team's performance. Within the context of these decisions, senior managers must consider the complexity of the organization and weigh the risks of keeping some staff against the dangers of going without the valuable information they have.

One chief executive took so much time assembling a new team that he left for another position fifteen months after he recruited the last executive. There was not enough time for him to implement his values and affect the culture of the organization. As a result, the CEO who followed him found the organization unwilling to take any risks or become excited with any of her initiatives.

Handling an Internal Promotion

Despite the difficulties involved in coming into a new organization, the challenges confronting senior managers who have been promoted from within an organization are also very great, and sometimes are even greater than for those coming from the outside. The newly promoted executive may be encumbered with excess baggage from past decisions and may have rivals or enemies looking for ways to undermine him or her. Internally promoted executives also frequently have difficulty assuming the authority of their new role.

Senior managers promoted from within should develop a number of themes that clearly build on past successes for the organization and should target specific areas for change. These themes might include organizational initiatives toward quality improvement or cost-effectiveness, changes in the organizational structure, or efforts to improve relations with medical staff.

Newly promoted executives also should emphasize their intimate knowledge of the organization and their ability to move the organization ahead quickly without losing any momentum. Of course, if the institution is in such a state of disarray that total turnaround is needed, then themes that emphasize stability and continuity will not work. Instead, the newly promoted executive will need to introduce themes of change and renewal.

Executives who have been promoted from within should also exercise extreme caution if others approach them about past promises and deals made by the previous executive. This is not the time to feel forced into actions that may not be beneficial. Ideally, these issues can be cleared up in the interview process by clarifying with the hiring authority so that the newly hired executive may begin with a clean slate.

Taking Leave

Senior executives should consider how to take leave when they determine that it is time to move on to other opportunities. Senior executives should consider whether they are running *away* from their jobs or *toward* other more attractive jobs. Although this may seem like a subtle difference, it is an important one. Some employers do not like to hire executives who are on the rebound and coming from a negative situation. Many employers prefer to seek out applicants in positive situations and recruit them away. This raises the issues of competence and fit, as well as timing. Most search consultants would agree that the best executives usually are not actively looking for new positions; they tend to believe that they can improve situations where they presently serve, and they usually are satisfied with their ongoing progress. This is not to say that these executives do not occasionally look for *bigger* opportunities or positions with more authority, responsibility, and greater variety. They seem to have a sense of when to look and when to respond to inquiries about their interest in other positions. Good people seldom find themselves in the position of having to leave bad situations because of their sense of timing.

Other executives (perhaps less effective ones) seem to be constantly looking for an easier position or one with fewer hassles. Others just seem to always be looking for a new job. These persons may not quite fit in either their particular positions or in health care in any position.

Senior managers and executives considering a change should try to figure out in which category they belong. They may need more than a change in venue with the same or similar responsibilities; they may need to consider a change in career or industry.

Executives should learn to determine when it is time to move on. Some senior managers seem to be flexible enough to change with each succeeding chief executive officer and to provide continuing value to their organization, but many do not seem able to read signs that suggest that it is time for them to leave. These signs might include seeing peer executives gain additional responsibilities while you do not, a shift in assignments resulting in a decrease in your authority or span of control, or reaching a plateau when few new initiatives or improvements can be made.

When a new chief executive joins an organization, all of the senior managers should take stock and assess their worth to the organization. They should also assess the style and values of the new leader and attempt to determine how or whether they fit well with them. This may be the time to prepare to move on.

The following protocols can help senior managers who are moving from one organization to another take leave successfully.

Do Not Burn Any Bridges

Executives leaving their jobs should not burn any bridges. The people left behind may be needed as allies and supporters in the future. For example, a chief human resources officer who resigned after ten years to begin a new job in another city determined after the first two weeks that the new job did not suit him. Because he had not burned his bridges, his former employer welcomed him back, and he continued to work for the hospital for another twenty years until retirement.

Another senior executive, when leaving an organization, said many negative things about peer executives. Two jobs later, the executive found that one of the former colleagues he had maligned was a senior vice president in the holding company of the hospital for which he worked.

In another example, a chief operating officer was not pleased that another senior executive, who reported to the chief executive officer, was leaving. The COO did not attend any of the departing executive's farewell parties and offered no words of congratulation. The COO was later interested in the chief operating officer position at this senior executive's new organization. Despite what seemed to be positive conversations about the position with this former teammate, he never was invited for an interview. The COO's poor manners during the senior executive's departure may have had something to do with his not being invited to interview.

Leave Graciously

Senior managers should be as gracious and appreciative as possible of the opportunity they have had to serve in the organization they are leaving. Valuable experiences are gained at any organization. Executives should not act as though they cannot wait to leave their present positions and begin their new jobs. While they are still on an organization's payroll, they are ethically bound to focus on that organization's issues and problems.

Leave Everything in Order

Senior managers who are leaving a position should take care to leave their affairs in order. They should prepare for their successor a memo outlining any outstanding matters, with recommendations for future action. Files should be well organized, and departing executives should discuss their contents with secretaries or other appropriate staff.

Managers should leave for their successors specific, detailed written performance evaluations of all their staff.

If it looks as though a subordinate will be promoted to replace the departing executive, the executive should be proud and do everything possible to prepare the person for his or her new position.

Departing managers should not take items belonging to the institution. It is appropriate to make copies of documents that are not confidential and do not contain proprietary information, but the originals must remain with the organization. Books purchased by the organization should remain there. Executives should carefully label any books that they personally purchased while at the organization.

Summary

A crucial time in an executive's career is when he or she first takes over a new position. The protocols for how to act and behave in such situations are essential to success. Senior managers and executives should carefully consider all that they say and do so that their first several months are carefully planned and orchestrated to maximize success.

Note

1. American College of Healthcare Executives, American Hospital Association, Heidrick and Struggles, *Hospital CEO Turnovers: 1981–1990* (Chicago: American College of Healthcare Executives, 1991).

17

IN THE OFFICE

Senior managers probably spend two-thirds of their waking time each week in the office. This is where they experience most of their career highs and lows and where they develop a sense of identity. The executive's office becomes an extension of his or her personality and style. Executives work hard to feel at home in their offices. Many try to make the office as relaxed and comfortable as possible as a trade-off for the many long hours spent at work.

However, this drive to create a homelike atmosphere at the office may be counterproductive. This book attempts to address many problems caused by senior managers getting *too* comfortable with their positions, status, power, and authority. This high comfort level may cause them to develop careless, sloppy work habits. Although it is appropriate and perhaps often necessary to be relaxed in one's position, it should not be taken to extremes. Careless, lackadaisical practices in the workplace can lead to inattentive, slipshod work. Executives who get too comfortable in their surroundings may risk exposure to many of the hazards described in this book.

The power of the office is often misunderstood and overlooked. To the subordinate, the executive's office represents his or her great power and influence. One midwestern hospital held an open house for its new executive offices and found that the chief executive's office was one of the most popular stops during the tour. The chief executive offered employees the opportunity to sit in his chair; those who did talked about it for weeks afterward. The employees came to see what they would have described as an inner sanctum, a place that is generally off-limits to them. This "ivory tower" aspect of the executive suite has a tremendous aura for most staff. To others, the executive office evokes fear and intimidation because of the power associated with the person who occupies the office.

Senior managers should consider protocols for:

1. General behavior in the office
2. Receiving people in the office
3. Officemates and office politics
4. Working with a secretary

General Office Protocols

Humor

An office is a place for work, not a club for trying out new comedy material. Senior managers should remember that in trying to develop and maintain an image, humor, while it has its place, can if used too often damage an executive's professional image. Some humor is suitable and fitting, but executives should exercise judgment in its use. Humor is appropriate if it is tasteful, if it does not demean others, and if it does not make fun of those in a less fortunate situation. Humor should not be used so much that the serious nature of the business atmosphere is disrupted.

Ethnic or off-color jokes are never appropriate in the office. They do not help get any job done, they can offend others and hurt morale, and they can damage senior managers' professional images. It is better to draw an absolute line on this and not risk insulting or hurting someone else.

One chief financial officer told off-color jokes around the senior secretaries and actually offended two of them so much that they eventually transferred to other positions within the organization. He did not know why this happened. Although the CFO's behavior would be considered sexual harassment under present employment discrimination laws, the two employees transferred rather than filing complaints.

This counsel does not mean that senior managers should not have and display a sense of humor. In fact, a sense of humor is one of the more important characteristics of a successful executive. However, it is important to keep it appropriate and balanced with the pressing demands of the organization.

Never Borrow Money from Coworkers

Executives should not borrow money from coworkers; it will be very damaging to the working relationship if the executive forgets or is unable to repay the loan. Both the borrower and the lender are put in uncomfortable positions when money is owed.

Respect Company Property

An office is owned by the corporation; it is not *personal* property. Therefore, senior managers should observe corporate restrictions. For example, if smoking is not permitted within the organization, they should not smoke in their offices. They should carefully care for the furniture and personal equipment in the office and be aware that others may use it someday.

Although it is appropriate to customize one's office to reflect personal style and preference, executives should not take this to extremes. For example, displaying personal trophies, awards, or family photographs may be quite acceptable, but it should be kept within reason. One midwestern CEO displayed over ten mounted fish in his office, along with several pictures of his hunting and fishing trips. At home, a person may have a favorite well-worn chair, but it is not suitable to have such a chair in the office setting.

Respect Traditions

When senior managers share an office suite with other executives and secretaries, they should follow the customs and traditions unless they have sound business reasons for doing otherwise. For example, if the custom for birthdays is for the celebrant to bring in his or her own cake, executives should be certain to do so; to fail to do so sends the message that one is rude and uncaring. (In some organizations, the chief executive officer may be exempt from such office traditions.)

Be cognizant of support-staff and peer-level office issues. There may be times when senior managers should refrain from joining the customs and traditions of the secretarial support staff. At other times the culture of the office may be such that senior managers should join in. Each executive suite has a personality of its own. As new senior managers join the staff, they must survey the practices, determine what seems right and wrong, and act accordingly.

A chief executive who comes into an office with well-established customs should exercise caution before trying to change them. It is appropriate to make some changes, but the executive should not make unreasonable mandates.

When one chief executive arrived at his new hospital, he found that the secretaries and the other senior managers in the executive suite had a monthly potluck lunch. The executive participated the first two months on the job but he then determined that these lunches sent an unintended message of inappropriate laxness and festiveness to the rest of the hospital. On the day of the potluck, food odors permeated the executive suite and wafted into the surrounding areas, and the atmosphere in the suite was relaxed and festive. The secretaries spent much of the morning preparing for the lunch and much of the afternoon cleaning up. A couple of visitors made comments to the chief executive that made him understand that they viewed this as unprofessional. In ending the tradition, the chief executive was careful to give a detailed explanation of his reasons and suggested that he and the other executives contribute to a similar gathering at a local restaurant on the fourth Friday of each month. Over the years, this event became very popular with the staff and enhanced morale in the executive suite.

The reader may ask: what is wrong with doing things that are helpful in developing and maintaining morale and spirit? Nothing, if they are appropriate activities that do not interfere with the smooth, timely conducting of business and they do not give a negative impression. This protocol does not suggest that if these or similar practices exist they should *always* be eliminated. New managers should consider the degree of formality in the community, the organization, and the executive suite. Generally speaking, it is important to maintain an environment of professionalism. Senior managers must recognize how office activities and customs appear to others and plan accordingly.

Maintaining a Professional Atmosphere in the Executive Suite

Executives should consider how the following situations affect the overall atmosphere in the executive suite:

- When the coffee room in the back of the executive suite is unkempt and littered with dishes, towels, and other sundry items, this gives a bad impression. Each person should clean up after himself or herself.

- When the executive office is in disarray, cluttered, or has trash that has not been picked up, this gives a bad impression.

- When the degree of informality becomes excessive within the executive suite, this decreases the image of competence presented to outsiders and other employees. Informality approaches the excessive level when it disrupts routine business conversations and focuses attention on non-work-related issues.

- When secretaries bring lunch in (which is quite often the case in many health care executive suites because of the fast pace), food odors may disturb the rest of the suite. Managers should consider providing a well-ventilated lunch area to better contain food odors. Of course, any leftovers should be properly disposed of and the lunch area should be kept clean.

These issues may seem minor, but they are part of developing an overall professional look and feel in the executive suite.

Do Not Fund-Raise in the Office

Executives must realize the power in their positions. Even though secretarial and other support staff may appear to really want to buy the executive's raffle tickets or participate in other fund-raising activities, they may in fact feel obligated to do so. Executives should avoid any fund-raising activities in the office.

Receiving People in the Office

Although much of the work done in the office is done privately, others, from both inside and outside the organization, will frequently use the facilities. Many of the protocols already presented in this book are useful in these situations, but there are several that have specific application here.

Receive People on Time

Executives should be on time for all appointments. If busy executives fill the short period between appointments by making or returning phone calls, they should be careful to end the calls in enough time to avoid receiving people with appointments late. Some senior managers may believe that by making a person wait they are showing power and authority. However, this is never appropriate behavior. If scheduled meetings tend to run into one another, senior managers and executives should consider spacing these meetings over a wider time period.

Treat Guests with Courtesy

Anyone who comes to a senior manager or executive's office as a visitor is a guest and should be treated accordingly. Be certain to offer the standard amenities, such as coffee or tea, and show the utmost professional courtesy.

Neatness Counts

A neat office not only aids personal time management but also gives a positive impression to visitors. Executives who work with large amounts of paper should consider ways to organize paper clutter (such as file folders) or store papers in areas other than where visitors are received to improve office tidiness.

Officemates and Office Politics

The principles discussed in Chapter 9 should be combined with the protocols described below.

Most organizations have senior-level managers working together in a confined space. These peers often spend more waking time together in the work setting than they do with their families. In many executive suites the group members try to develop a personal closeness, spending time together in social settings outside the office. Their families may socialize together. These social gatherings for most senior executives are a strong cog in the machinery of team building. Organizations need a strong, cohesive senior team to move successfully forward. Informal social gatherings are often substituted for well-planned team-building exercises with targeted goals and strategies designed to involve all members of the team.

As a result of these gatherings, however, several things can happen that can unglue or harm the team.

- Group members can become *too* comfortable with one another and develop an excessive degree of informality that is carried back to the workplace. This can be counterproductive when the group deals with difficult issues, because the informality will often surface at inappropriate times. For example, joking about a weekend party during a team meeting may be disruptive and inappropriate.

- Some group members may form cliques that can be destructive back at the office. These groups will often plan their strategies in social settings and seem conspiratorial in the workplace.

- Some spouses of peer executives within the organization may form especially close friendships and share information heard in confidence, which can have damaging results for other team members. When these alliances surface at work they can cause divisions within the team.

- Some spouses do not feel comfortable attending such events and many may not want to attend all of them. If the executive does not go without his or her spouse, he or she may lose out as a result of not being a part of the social scene.

- Spouses may be uncertain about what they should or should not say at these events or how they should behave. They may be fearful that their statements or behavior might have a negative effect on their spouse's reputation or authority at work. Some may talk too freely about information that should be confidential; others may bring up inappropriate information about team divisiveness or team problems.

It is naive to believe that these issues can be totally avoided. However, this is an area where senior managers and executives should be most careful. They may wish to avoid discussions of particularly sensitive topics with their spouses, or they may try to clearly delineate those issues that are highly confidential and off-limits for discussion outside the family. As a final effort to minimize risk in social settings, many organizations use calculated team-building efforts and will either choose to avoid poorly planned social gatherings or will develop them with very specific purposes in mind.

Personal Relationships with Subordinate Managers

The chief executive should carefully consider how to provide off-hours socializing opportunities for the senior team. Although it is appropriate to spend time out of the office trying to get to know one another on a more personal basis, these events are still business get-togethers. Executives' behavior, while relaxed, should be professional.

Chief executives must be cautious not to create the perception that some team members have greater access to them than others. If this apparent access seems to be the result of outside opportunities to socialize, it can be destructive to office morale.

An imperfect line often must be drawn between chief executives and their subordinate executives, particularly when it comes to friendships. Chief executives must remember that they have ultimate authority in their organizations. In reality, friendships that are not based on the equal footing of both parties cannot be easily maintained. It is indeed lonely at the top, and friendships, while possible between people at different levels within the workplace, are very difficult to maintain.

Working with a Secretary

Senior managers' secretaries can be assets *or* liabilities. Prior to beginning a discussion on working with secretaries, two important points must be made.

First, many of the protocols that follow are predicated upon the assumption that senior managers are working in organizations where they are not owners but rather employees of the organizations. What is the difference? There may be situations where a secretary working directly for an *owner* will be required to undertake as part of the conditions of employment certain personal duties. In these situations some of the protocols suggested here may not be appropriate.

In organizations where senior managers are employees, not owners, those senior managers must always keep in mind that their secretaries work *for the organization* and *not for them.* It is not appropriate to expect a secretary to perform personal tasks such as typing the boss' personal tax returns, running personal errands, or handling correspondence for members of the family not employed with the organization.

Second, the relationship between senior executives and their secretaries should be *professional*, not personal. This is particularly important when the senior manager is male and the secretary is female. There must always be due diligence to avoid the perception that the relationship has become *too* personal.

Although their secretaries are very important to senior managers, many act as though secretaries have little value and are simply "office equipment," like the word processor. Although many executives claim to value their secretaries, few act as if they do. The degree of respect an executive shows a secretary often can predict how beneficial the secretary can be to the executive.

Share Information with Secretaries

Executives should inform secretaries of the rationales and reasons behind decisions, discuss with them the direction of the organization and areas of responsibilities, and provide them with background information on some of the current issues. Such secretaries can later provide better backup in the absence of executives and are likely to become informed supporters of their policies.

Secretaries Are Not Servants

Some things are appropriate for executives to ask their secretaries to do; others are inappropriate. Secretaries should not be asked to perform such personal tasks such as balancing the executives' personal checkbook, buying gifts for their spouses, placing personal telephone calls, picking up laundry, or handling chores for their children.

There may be some exceptions to this rule. For example, when a senior manager has returned late from a meeting and is due to go to another meeting and drops her automobile off in front of the building, it may be appropriate for her to ask her secretary to park it. There are a number of other possible exceptions; however, it is always best to err on the side of conservatism.

Along these same lines is the question of who makes and gets the coffee. Senior managers are probably acting appropriately when they ask their secretaries to prepare and serve coffee or other drinks for guests in the executive suite. However, senior managers should not take advantage of their secretaries in this way and should certainly make and pour their own coffee when they are alone.

The same issue arises when busy senior managers and executives ask their secretaries to get them lunch so that they can work through lunch. In these situations, it may be quite appropriate for senior managers to ask their secretaries to pick up their lunches, but they should not make a habit of asking their secretaries to handle these requests as though they were personal servants. Executives should also consider returning the favor by offering to pick up lunch for secretaries who are unable to get away for their meal.

A good general rule is that secretaries can be asked to get coffee or lunch or to help in other ways as a favor or as a courtesy but *not* as a condition of employment. The boss should also close the circle by returning the courtesy. Executives should show good judgment, avoid appearing sexist, and act respectful to secretaries.

Show Common Courtesy

Executives should strive to be courteous at all times with their secretaries. There is a tendency for senior managers to become too informal and relaxed with secretaries who are long-time employees. Even routine interpersonal exchanges should be made with the utmost courtesy. This guideline helps to keep the relationship on a professional level that others can respect.

Focus on Work

Senior managers and executives should focus the working relationship on work-related expectations. Maintain regularly scheduled sessions to set forth specific work expectations. This helps to concentrate the boss-secretary relationship on work rather than on personal issues.

Executives should keep discussions of personal affairs and issues out of the office. If secretaries bring up issues that might be deemed too personal, senior managers should change the subject; this will convey that they are not comfortable discussing a personal subject.

This protocol may be particularly useful in situations where the executive or secretary is going through a separation or divorce from a spouse. Personal discussions about the details of such a situation can harm the professional working relationship. If the line between business and personal issues has been appropriately drawn from the start of the relationship, then there is a greater ability to keep it out of the conversation later.

Misperceptions Can Be Damaging

Male senior managers in particular should be aware of possible misperceptions when they and their female secretaries go out to lunch together. The grapevines in most organizations are all too likely to create false rumors that can be damaging to careers or success within the organization.

Any Physical Contact Is Risky

Never touch secretaries (or other subordinates). This includes pats on the back and affectionate arms around the shoulder. Although these physical expressions may be well-intentioned and innocent, they could be misinterpreted by either the secretary or by anyone else who might be watching.

Behave Courteously When Sharing a Secretary

There are often situations where several executives share the same suite and the same secretary. In such situations, executives should be careful not to monopolize the secretary's time. Executives should coordinate their workloads so that conflicting priorities do not unfairly impose upon the secretary.

Do Not Assume That Secretaries Know What Is Confidential

Executives should not assume that a secretary knows what is confidential and what is not. They should clearly identify any information that they want their secretaries to keep confidential.

Clarify Expectations

Senior managers often make the unfair assumption that secretaries know exactly what is expected of them. They should be certain to spell out what they expect of their secretaries, and they should set aside time to listen to what their secretaries expect of them. The two must work together as a team, and the two most important elements of effective teams are the agreement and understanding of goals and the negotiation of roles and expectations. Such issues as when it is necessary to work though lunch or stay late or work over a weekend should be clearly spelled out.

Do Not Give Overly Personal Gifts

The exchange of overly personal gifts between a boss and a secretary is inappropriate. Even such items as gloves, scarves, or cologne can be subject to misinterpretation; these kinds of personal gifts put the focus of the relationship into a *personal* rather than a business arena.

Appropriate gifts include food items, books (on topics that are not overly personal), items for the office, or gift certificates at department stores. The key is to keep gifts reasonable and suitable.

Gifts for secretaries should not be expensive. An expensive gift might send the unintended message that the cost of the gift is a measure of the boss's appreciation. Also, expensive gifts may make the secretary feel obligated to try to match the expense of the gift. Secretaries should be discouraged from spending a great deal on gifts for their bosses. Perhaps the executive could ask that a donation be made to a favorite charity instead. All gifts should be given discreetly at a time when others will not be present.

Summary

The office is the setting for an executive's work life. Many of the protocols presented in this chapter are matters of personal judgment and should not be viewed as absolutes. Many variables affect the approach a senior manager or executive should take. It is hoped that this chapter has gotten readers to focus on potential pitfalls in the very area where they may feel most comfortable—the executive suite. To coin a phrase that might be applicable here, "comfort brings concern and possible danger." Successful executives tend not to let their guard down. They tend to be aware of how things appear to others and they are sensitive to how others expect things to look within a professional office setting.

18

DIVERSITY IN THE WORKPLACE

Diversity is a hallmark of the United States, and the employee population of health care facilities reflects this. Usually diversity refers to the diverse racial and cultural groups that make up the U.S. work force, and U.S. society in general. Most of the issues surrounding this theme and those that are covered in the greatest detail in this chapter pertain to this dimension. However, in its strictest sense, diversity simply means "being different." It incorporates not only race and culture, but also age, physical abilities, gender, and sexual orientation. As executives consider how they relate to others within and outside of the workplace, the issue of diversity will surface time and again. One of the greatest leadership challenges today is how to deal with this increasing diversity.

One of the most difficult concerns about diversity is the conflict between the desire to assimilate those who are diverse within the mainstream of the organization and the desire of those who are diverse to maintain all or some of their diversity. Obviously, much of this is a challenge to society in general and cannot be adequately addressed within this book. Nonetheless, senior managers and executives should be aware of this ongoing conflict. Marilyn Loden and Judy B. Rosener, in *Workforce America: Managing Employee Diversity as a Vital Resource*, describe the friction this way: "This focus on changing diverse people has created difficulties for many people of color, women, differently abled, gay, and ethnically diverse people who want to maintain their own cultural heritages as they move ahead in their careers. For while such individuals can often maintain their diverse identities at the entry level, the range of acceptable behavior narrows as one moves up the career ladder."[1]

The protocols in this book target appropriate behavior and suggest certain standards and other principles that executives should follow because of the demands placed upon them by society and their organizations. Certain conduct is suggested because it probably will be helpful in one's career. However, increasing diversity in the work force may lead to some modifications. For example, one standard of personal hygiene in U.S. culture is fresh breath. Should someone from a culture that favors spicy food with lots of garlic be expected to follow this standard of garlic-free breath?

Much of this chapter is directed at a health care leadership circle that is predominantly from a white Anglo culture; to date, a great proportion of the senior leaders of U.S. health care come from this group. An underlying theme, however, is that the population that is served by these individuals and the employee population working within their organizations are becoming much more diverse. Changes will occur at the top both in terms of sensitivity of senior management to issues of diversity and in terms of the composition of senior management itself. This transformation will be neither quick nor simple; it will require the skillful guidance of those leaders who clearly comprehend the need to embrace and incorporate the increasing diversity of the workplace.

Although, as was mentioned above, most persons think of diversity in terms of *racial* and *cultural* differences, there is a need to consider *all kinds of differences*. Those who are different in any way fit the category of diversity. Dealing effectively with diversity may mean how well one relates to a file clerk who has a hearing deficiency; it may call for more progressive methods of working with those who have other kinds of handicaps; it may call for greater tolerance of different concepts of society, institutions, and so-called social norms.

Workforce 2000

The work force that senior health care managers face now and will face in the future is one of increasing diversity. Most of this diversity is racial and cultural. The Hudson Institute's now-famous study, *Workforce 2000: Work and Workers for the 21st Century*, is must reading for all health care executives.

There are three notable findings in this study. The first is that minorities will comprise the most significant numbers of new entrants to the work force. According to *Workforce 2000*, "non-whites will make up 29 percent of the new entrants into the labor force between now and the year 2000, twice their current share of the work force."[2]

The second is that "immigrants will represent the largest share of the increase in the population and the workforce since the first World War."[3] It is expected that a large number of these immigrants will be of working age and will go into the work force. Since the publishing of *Workforce 2000* in 1987, the collapse of the Berlin Wall and the easing of government controls in former Communist countries have made it likely that immigration to the United States will increase. They have also increased the likelihood that traditions and institutional customs that were once held sacrosanct will be increasingly challenged in the future. Not only will the issue of diversity be a challenge in terms of the different groups of people in the work force, but it will also increase the likelihood that people will confront and contest much of what organizations hold dear.

Third, the Hudson Institute reported that by the year 2000, women will make up about 47 percent of the work force. A largely female work force is nothing new for health care, but there will continue to be an impact as women move into fields that previously were dominated by men. Health care employers may be hard-hit by women's defection.

Working Woman magazine gave an excellent summary of the Hudson Institute's findings. Audrey Edwards wrote in the January 1991 issue, "It is clearly no longer a man's world, and certainly not a white man's world, given that he is expected to account for only 32 percent of the entering work force by 2000."[4]

This chapter will not present a lengthy discourse on these demographic factors. It will suggest to senior managers and executives that there are sound reasons to prepare for a vastly changed work force over the next few years. Management in this country historically has not done a very effective job of dealing with diversity. Senior management (which consists predominantly of white males) and employers in all industries historically have lacked the sensitivity and insight needed to appropriately deal with minority groups. The many equal employment opportunity laws and the numerous claims of employment discrimination validate this claim.

The senior executives who will be best equipped to deal with a diverse work force will be those who learn the customs and characteristics of the different groups in the world of work. They will use this knowledge to better understand that each group consists of people whose differences are acceptable in the workplace.

For some, this chapter will discuss issues they have already dealt with in the past; some areas of the country, such as New York, Miami, Chicago, and Los Angeles, already have health care work forces that are very diverse. For others, these issues may be new considerations because they have not been exposed to diversity in the work force and the challenges it brings.

The Baby Bust

The "baby bust" is another factor that will play a major role in the health care workplace of the future. The facts are simple: there will be fewer young people to fill entry-level positions and enter college programs that are feeder systems for the health care field. Furthermore, a large number of health care workers who have worked in the same entry-level jobs for twenty-five to thirty years are retiring in increasing numbers. With the resulting labor shortages, the scarcity of qualified applicants will give the remaining applicants more bargaining power. Minorities and members of other groups (such as the physically challenged) who now have some difficulty entering the work force will become more valuable. Because of the pressure to fill positions resulting from the shortage of entry-level labor, the power and status of all minorities and the differently abled will increase. They will be more attracted to employers whose management is prepared to cope positively with their diversity.

One final note is in order at this point. Much of this chapter deals with the tension between races, particularly between whites and African Americans. This is the area that presents the most challenge for our society. Although there have been many increases in employment and other opportunities for African Americans (as well as other ethnic minorities), there remains a tension between the races. George Davis and Gregg Watson discuss their concern about this in *Black Life in Corporate America: Swimming in the Mainstream*. They consider it disturbing that within the workplace, race is seldom a topic of conversation. As they put it, "On the surface blacks and whites get along quite well in most corporate settings. They don't seem to mind working with each other. They laugh together and call each other 'friend.' However, blacks are often oppressed by this silence on race. Their careers and morale are affected by this thing that they cannot mention."[5]

There is much work yet to be done in this area. By improving our ability to cope with racial issues, we will also learn valuable lessons that can be applied in all areas of diversity. Sensitivity, receptiveness to dissimilarity, and principles of mediation and compromise are applicable across all areas of diversity.

Protocols for a Diverse Work Force

How can senior managers and executives prepare to deal with a culturally diverse work force? The protocols described below will help this process.

Respect the Dignity of Others

Having respect for the dignity of others is the foundation of any efforts to work effectively with people from different cultures.

The other protocols in this chapter all evolve from this main protocol. Having respect for others requires a willingness to realize that one's own way is not necessarily the right and only way. It requires a healthy curiosity about other people, cultures, customs, and traditions. Senior managers and executives who are willing to learn about other people and customs display a true respect for others. They will be better able to adapt to the changes that will result from the increasing diversity of the work force.

There is an interesting side note here that pertains to a popular approach to patient relations and helps to illustrate the significance of respect. One well-known national consultant has suggested that those who deal with patients need only *act* as though they are happy to help patients. They do not have to *feel* happy about it. There are those who suggest that the same concept applies to dealing with employees from diverse cultural and ethnic groups. They point out that within the work setting, one does not have to actually *like* people from different cultural and ethnic groups but merely has to act *as though* one did. The problem with this approach is that it is insincere, and many people can detect the lack of genuine regard and esteem for them. If one thinks in terms of *respecting* rather than *liking* others, it becomes easier to treat people as individuals rather than generalizing about them based on customs or practices that are unfamiliar to us.

Practice True Acceptance, Not Just Quiet Tolerance

Although equal opportunity in the workplace may seem to have made great strides in the past several years, a more covert problem may have arisen that will create increasing difficulties for those who attempt to manage a work force of increasing cultural diversity. As was mentioned earlier, this covert problem is described by George Davis and Gregg Watson in *Black Life in Corporate America: Swimming in the Mainstream.* This study dealt with black managers who were working in corporations throughout the country. The authors (who are both African-American) state that "there are few instances in corporations where anyone is allowed to complain about the life in any significant way." They also say "we were concerned that within corporations there was not a great deal of talk about race. It is mentioned only when it becomes obvious that a racial problem must be dealt with. Subtle racial problems are ignored. Deep-seated ones are often treated as if they don't exist."[6]

There are many underlying problems between the different races and cultures that make up the work force—and the society. The first step for dealing with these difficulties is to develop open and sincere feelings of respect for those who are different. This respect must encompass an acceptance of the apparent differences and an awareness that these variations do not mean inferiority.

Learn about Other Cultures

Executives should learn about the different cultures and races in the organization. They should acquaint themselves with the issues and problems of importance to minority groups in the United States.

Practice Affirmative Action in Hiring

Senior managers should work hard to hire and promote minorities (including women) into management-level positions. This is not only good business in that it provides a middle management that is attuned to the special needs of a diverse work force, but it also shows that management has a true commitment to diversity. Furthermore, it provides senior-level managers with better insight into racial, cultural, and gender differences. However, this tactic often raises protests from whites (particularly white males). Their first thought is of quotas and pressures to hire a woman or a member of a minority group whether or not he or she is the best qualified.

Senior managers who have not had any open and serious conversations with members of minority groups on the meaning of the word "qualifications" may lack crucial information. To many minorities, the word "qualifications" is a code word that white managers use as an excuse to avoid hiring them. Many members of minority groups have not had sufficient opportunity to gain the education and experience to help them meet the qualifications for many positions.

Although hiring the most qualified candidate is a reasonable business expectation, senior managers should consider what qualifications are truly necessary to do the job. This is much less a science than an art. Using criteria that exclude minorities will ultimately harm the organization. If managers wish to become more adept at dealing with a culturally diverse work force, they should work aggressively toward the goal of employing more members of minority groups. Many community-based programs can help to integrate minorities into the work force through volunteer programs and internships.

Organizations that have worked aggressively to employ the differently abled in various positions also report remarkable positive returns. Even before the passage of the Americans with Disabilities Act (ADA) in 1992, a number of health care employers were successfully employing persons who were included in the ADA definition of handicapped. Effective executives will do well to investigate these opportunities with an open mind.

Celebrate Other Cultures

Senior managers and executives should encourage the organization to celebrate other cultures. One of the best ways to do this is to have a theme day in the hospital cafeteria and serve food from the particular culture being celebrated. A large number of hospitals throughout the country have had very favorable responses from employees (and visitors and patients) to such programs. Decorations and other items symbolic of the culture being celebrated can be displayed, which adds to the educational value as well as the festive atmosphere.

During January, executives may want to commemorate Dr. Martin Luther King's birthday by developing programs that focus on the meaning of his life and work. An assembly to which local leaders of the African American community are invited could be held to recognize his contributions. Some organizations have also invited local gospel choirs to perform during these programs.

Organizations with a large number of Asian Americans should consider holding programs that celebrate the various Asian cultures and customs. The same is true for organizations with large Latino populations.

Sponsor a Cultural Diversity Day

Executives may want to sponsor a Cultural Diversity Day that would not focus on any particular ethnic group or culture but instead would celebrate cultural diversity in general and would help all staff members to be sensitive to and appreciative of it. One hospital listed as many different employees as possible who were willing to identify their cultural backgrounds. This information was part of a display outside the cafeteria that bore the heading "We Are Proud of Our Heritage." A number of these employees provided personal stories of their grandparents and other relatives who had come to this country from other lands. This provided the organization an opportunity to see the vast size of the melting pot that existed there.

**Support Programs for Management of
Conflict and Cultural Harassment**

Executives should show personal support for programs that enhance the organization's ability (and willingness) to deal with conflict, particularly conflict involving cultural diversity. They should develop a formal program for conflict management within the human resources department to deal specifically with cultural conflict. Ideally, the organization should hire members of minority groups represented in the organization to work in the program. The program should include formal mechanisms to hear and address grievances emanating from cultural conflicts.

Organizations should also develop specific training programs that emphasize understanding of and sensitivity to the diverse cultural groups among their employees. These programs should address the degree to which the organization expects assimilation and the degree to which diversity will be embraced and fostered. Members of different minority groups should participate in the development and presentation of all of these programs. Senior managers should attend to show their genuine support for the programs.

Just as there is a need for meaningful training and education on dealing with sexual harassment in the workplace, there should also be programs that focus on racial and cultural harassment. Harassment in this respect includes telling culturally insensitive jokes and teasing or stereotyping people of a particular cultural or racial background.

Make Diversity a Part of Everyday Life

Senior managers should *talk* about cultural diversity in the organization and acclimate the work force to the fact that cultural diversity will increase and that it is an issue with which the organization must become familiar.

All managers should bring up the issue of cultural diversity in their own work groups. Perhaps certain senior managers could become active advocates for cultural diversity by keeping the team aware of diversity issues and challenges and by speaking up in support of hiring programs and educational offerings. Ideally the human resources executive should serve this role, although others could as well.

Try to Recruit Board Members from Diverse Cultures

Executives should work to develop cultural and ethnic diversity on the board of trustees. The board should mirror the community it serves.

Pay Attention to Physical Plant Issues

Senior executives should make sure that their organization's signage is sensitive to cultural and language issues. They might be surprised at the need for and positive response to multilingual signs. The physical plant must also meet the needs of the differently abled, through features such as Braille elevator buttons, wheelchair access, and special telephones for the hearing impaired.

Be Active in Community Programs that Address Cultural Diversity

Executives should be active in community programs, such as service clubs or community social agencies, that address cultural diversity. Consider an adopt-a-school program in which the institution works closely with area public schools that have a large number of students from racial or cultural minorities.

Senior managers should also welcome minority volunteers in their organizations. They should recruit minorities by appealing to minority leaders within the community for volunteers. The presence of minority volunteers will send a positive message to minorities in the community and will help them feel more comfortable as patients or visitors in the institution.

Finally, senior executives should offer organizational support to social and sports activities that involve members of diverse ethnic and cultural groups. Company-sponsored teams often are excellent mechanisms to get different races and cultures together and may enhance teamwork.

Summary

The workplace will change substantially within the coming few years. Increasing cultural divergence will present many new challenges to senior managers. Following the protocols discussed in this chapter and attempting to respect the dignity and diversity of others should help to develop and maintain a cooperative and peaceful workplace.

Notes

1. M. Loden and J. B. Rosener, *Workforce America: Managing Employee Diversity as a Vital Resource* (Homewood, IL: Business One Irwin, 1991), 34.
2. Hudson Institute, *Workforce 2000: Work and Workers for the 21st Century* (Indianapolis: Hudson Institute, 1987), 19.
3. Ibid., 20.
4. A. Edwards, "The Enlightened Manager: How to Treat All Your Employees Fairly," *Working Woman* (January 1991), 45.
5. G. Davis and G. Watson, *Black Life in Corporate America: Swimming in the Mainstream* (New York: Anchor Books/Doubleday, 1985), 2.
6. Ibid.

Further Reading

American College of Healthcare Executives and the National Association of Health Services Executives, *A Racial Comparison of Career Attainment in Healthcare Management: Findings of a National Survey of Black and White Healthcare Executives.* Research Series No. 4. Chicago: American College of Healthcare Executives, 1993.

19

MEN AND WOMEN IN THE WORKPLACE

There are many important issues related to men and women in the workplace. Health care has had a predominantly female work force for many years. There are many changes in society as a whole that affect senior managers and executives who are trying to practice appropriate behavior relative to gender differences.

It is important to note that there are many societal norms that contribute to certain double standards of behavior for men and women. Although awareness of and sensitivity to this has greatly increased over the past several years, the standards of conduct in most communities still foster certain expectations of women that do not exist for men. Ideally, over time, standards will become the same for both sexes and women will not have to obey two sets of rules.

Issues regarding gender differences make headlines and create strife within the workplace. Sexual harassment, pay inequities, the glass ceiling, and the "mommy track" are frequently discussed and sometimes hotly debated topics. Executives who aspire to effective leadership and professional success should learn appropriate protocols for dealing with gender differences.

Some basic facts about the health care industry reveal why managers in this field must consider how gender differences affect their work force and the workplace.

- Most (probably 78 to 82 percent) of the health care work force is female.

- Health care leadership is considered by many to be one of the strongest bastions of male dominance, given the high percentage of physicians and administrators who are male and nurses and support services staff who are female.

• However, health care has long contained a pocket of senior-level women executives—sisters from religious orders who run health care organizations. They provide a greater concentration of female senior-level leadership than in any other industry.

• The balance of power is shifting in health care as increasing numbers of women go into both the practice of medicine and health care administration.

• An increasing number of women are entering graduate programs of health care administration.

• Typical boards of trustees of health care organizations tend to be dominated by males, sometimes having only one seemingly token female. These boards also have tended to be very conservative.

These facts are combined with demographic factors affecting U.S. society as a whole that will have direct impact on the health care workplace. For example, increasing numbers of women are moving into the work force; more women are working outside the home than ever before; there are more career opportunities for women today than ever before.

Men and women work together in many different kinds of workplaces. In health care, however, some issues arise that do not exist in other industries. First, hospitals have many physicians who practice within the hospital but are not its employees. Although more woman physicians are joining the ranks, most are male. The physicians work with a predominantly female group of nurses. Because the physicians are not employees per se, there is not the usual employer control over the physicians that exists in other industries, where everybody in the work group is an employee. This dynamic only compounds the problems of sexual harassment and sexist attitudes that historically have occurred between a mostly male medical staff and a mostly female nursing staff.

Second, health care organizations usually have at least one female senior-level manager, the chief nursing officer. There are, of course, exceptions where the chief nursing officer may be male. However, even if all of the other senior managers are male, there is frequently at least this one female in their midst. Many other industries typically have no women at the senior management level.

With the many demographic changes in society, the influx of women into health care jobs that traditionally have been male-dominated, and the special aspects of the health care industry, senior managers and executives must be more acutely aware of their behaviors and actions as they relate to gender.

The future in health care may well see

- more female physicians than male;
- a majority of chief executive officers who are female;
- childcare centers in every health care center;
- job sharing by female physicians and other female health care workers;
- predominantly female boards of trustees; and
- many female chiefs of staff and department chairs.

There are some general protocols that should be considered when looking at how men and women work together in health care. They are presented here in the hope that both sexes can become more sensitive to gender-related issues. Having a sense of the appropriate is especially important in dealing with these issues.

Sexual Harassment

Sexual harassment is a serious issue and problem in the workplace today. In a sense it is unfortunate that as a result of federal laws regarding this behavior, the term *sexual harassment* was created, as this term seems to refer to overt or blatant behavior and to exclude so-called innocent comments or activity that may make people uncomfortable. In reality, though, the phrase refers to *all* forms of conduct and behavior that may make people feel threatened or uncomfortable because of their gender.

For many men, harassment connotes aggressive, hostile behavior that is malicious and injurious. Thus, many men who are accused of sexual harassment deny it vigorously because of their interpretation of the meaning of the phrase. The fact is, however, that no matter what it is called, many women within the workplace do not feel comfortable with behaviors, actions, words, and looks that are sexual in nature. Men may claim that these cause no harm, but they are nonetheless inappropriate and wrong.

For the purposes of this chapter, sexual harassment means any behavior or attitude that makes people feel degraded, demeaned, or threatened because of their gender and any action or attention relating to gender that people find unwelcome. Interestingly, the law states that an action or behavior is not necessary to create a condition of sexual harassment. If even the atmosphere in which one works is uncomfortable because of sexual issues, then a condition of harassment exists. Although most of this discussion targets sexual harassment that is initiated by males against females, the opposite can (and does) occur.

Besides being illegal, sexual harassment can be an explosive issue for senior managers, as the following examples show.

Example A

A male administrator had worked successfully at a western hospital for three years when he began a relationship with his secretary. The relationship started very slowly and built eventually into a full-blown sexual affair. The obvious romance was a frequent topic of conversation in the organization. As the secretary became aware of the notoriety of the romance, she believed it was in the best interest of both parties to break it off. However, the man did not want to do so. As a result of her distancing herself from him, their relationship in the workplace suffered. He began to push her harder and harder and demanded unreasonable work output from her. He criticized her in front of others and gave her a negative performance appraisal. Eventually she went to the medical staff president to discuss her concern. Within six months, the board asked the administrator to leave. The secretary stayed on and successfully served the next two administrators.

Example B

A male chief financial officer at a midwestern hospital found new computer software that could print out drawings of large-busted women. He took one of these printouts into an office full of women and showed it to them, asking: "Don't you all wish that you looked like this?" The incident was reported to the CEO, who severely reprimanded the CFO and asked him to make a public apology. The CFO suffered a serious loss of credibility and influence.

Example C

A young male administrator in an eastern hospital had a young, attractive secretary. He often would comment on her looks, complimenting her on her clothing or hair or aspects of her appearance. On the surface, his comments were quite innocent; none of his remarks were sexually explicit, and his intent in making the comments was merely to be complimentary. However, the secretary considered the statements to be sexual in nature. She was offended and complained to his boss that she felt very uncomfortable working for him. After a long discussion with his boss about this, the assistant administrator ceased these kinds of comments. However, his working relationship with his secretary was never the same again. This young executive later left the organization, feeling that his professional effectiveness had been greatly harmed by the stiff relationship that existed between him and his secretary.

Protocols for Men and Women in the Workplace

Each of the examples described above is an example of sexual harassment. The executives could have avoided the negative impact on their personal and professional lives if they had followed the protocols described below, which are aimed at avoiding or dealing with sexual harassment.

Follow a Strict Hands-Off Rule

Senior managers and executives should keep their hands to themselves. Any touch other than a handshake runs the risk of misinterpretation. Executives who put their arms around others or pat them affectionately risk having such touches misconstrued by others as sexual advances. Senior managers should discipline themselves so that not touching others becomes second nature. Even if the person being touched does not consider the touches to be sexual in nature, the touches are inappropriate if the person is made uncomfortable by them. Subordinates may be hesitant to tell senior managers that the touches make them uncomfortable.

Avoid Looks that Carry Sexual Messages

Executives, male or female, must avoid giving "looks that undress"; that is, looks that carry sexual connotations. Such looks are totally inappropriate within the workplace.

Avoid Discussions and Dialogues of a Sexual Nature

Avoid entirely any discussions with any sexual references. This includes any reference to sexual differences as well as gender-oriented humor. The workplace is not a place for sexual jokes or innuendoes. It is not worth the risk to tell even a seemingly mild joke of a sexual nature.

Handle Sexual Harassment Professionally

Federal law mandates that organizations must have a means of dealing with charges of sexual harassment. Unfortunately, in many organizations it is merely a seldom-followed written policy. Senior managers should create within their own areas of responsibility a formal mechanism for dealing with charges of sexual harassment.

Senior managers and executives should take charges of sexual harassment very seriously, but they should also consider the possibility that the charges are false. Charges should be put in writing and senior managers should ascertain whether the party making the charge is willing to formally pursue the matter. If that person is willing, senior managers should conduct a formal investigation of the facts, taking into consideration the seriousness and gravity of the behavior. Where appropriate senior managers should take disciplinary action that matches the seriousness of the behavior.

Senior executives should send strong messages that they will not tolerate sexual harassment. There should be an attitude within the organization that encourages the airing of sexual grievances. The workplace is not an area for immature sexual behavior. Senior managers and executives can enhance their reputations and their leadership ability by handling sexual harassment issues effectively.

Avoid Dangerous Misperceptions

Senior managers and executives should watch very closely how they behave with persons of the opposite sex. It is advisable that managers not go out alone for lunch with their secretaries (or any subordinate) of the opposite sex. During National Secretaries Week, for example, another manager and secretary should join the two. The emphasis here is on secretaries because that is a relationship that traditionally has caused rumors in many organizations. The same possibility of misperception exists whenever a man and woman go out of the building for lunch or an outside meeting.

Senior managers and executives must always be aware of the appearance of impropriety. They should consider what others might think when they see a manager arriving at and leaving the workplace with a person of the opposite sex. This does not suggest that this should never happen, but simply that it can look suspicious and may stimulate gossip. Many potentially compromising situations are unavoidable. The best guideline is to ensure that they do not happen on a regular basis with the same people.

Use Discretion When Traveling on Business

Business travel with a person of the opposite sex can invite rumors and supposition. Senior managers should try to modify arrangements if possible (for example, have three or more individuals on the same trip). If this is not possible, then they should be fully aware of possible misperceptions. Managers should avoid making these trips on a regular basis.

Be Cautious When Working Late

Senior managers and executives should beware of negative perceptions if they occasionally work late with persons of the opposite sex (especially secretaries). A simple suggestion is to avoid leaving the building together after working late.

Morality is not the issue here; the issue is the perceptions of others and what may result organizationally from talk and innuendoes. Executives' ability to anticipate and manage other people's perceptions is the key to dealing with this potential problem. If many employees in the organization perceive that senior managers are having sexual affairs with other employees, the managers must deal with that perception, true or false. Something that is done in all innocence can be misconstrued and distorted, causing senior managers and subordinates great harm.

Leave Early

When a senior manager or executive joins a group of men and women to go out socially (for example, for drinks after work), he or she should avoid being among the last to leave the gathering. In addition, a man and a woman should avoid leaving together. Perception is more important than reality.

Male-Female Relationships

The ideal is that there should be no romantic relationships in the workplace when one or both parties hold management positions. This may seem harsh and may ignore the fact of life that people meet and fall in love, but this book is targeted at getting senior managers and executives to eliminate the kinds of behavior that can create obstacles in their pursuit of professional success and effectiveness. This is one area where senior managers and executives can try to avoid potential problems by exercising self-discipline.

The term *relationship* as used here describes a broad range of romantic involvement, from dating to marriage or cohabitation. Harsh and stern as it may seem, there are things that people must sacrifice when they move into management and particularly senior management, and romantic alliances with coworkers fall into that category.

Why is this "social abstinence" necessary? Consider the following reasons:

- When two people have a relationship and one is or both are in management roles, it almost always creates an overall negative perception about what that relationship means to the organization.

- There is the risk that others will perceive that there is favoritism in the distribution of resources, trading of corporate secrets, an unfair advantage being offered by the relationship, the conspiring against others, and biased professional judgments.

- Personal disputes between the parties may be brought into the workplace and negatively affect business there.

- Others in the workplace may find it very difficult to be direct and candid to one partner about the other.

- By keeping relationships out of the workplace, the problem of what to do if one person in the partnership is successful in the organization and one is not is avoided.

- Unequal pay, responsibility, and recognition can cause problems.

- Couples can become too informal with each other within the workplace.

- The office gossip within an organization can have a negative effect on productivity.

- There is the possibility that the productivity of the two parties in the romance will decline as they become preoccupied with each other.

People will continue to meet and be attracted to one another in the workplace. They will sometimes begin to socialize more intimately and may fall in love. If these natural occurrences transpire and if senior managers are involved, they should at least be aware of possible consequences.

Working Women—Equals with Men

Women may be very different from men in many respects; however, in the workplace, those differences should be insignificant. If a woman has unique skills, knowledge, or abilities that might be considered related to gender, she should use the skills, but she should not point them out in an obvious way. Similarly, a man should not call attention to gender-related characteristics. Managers should avoid any outward suggestion of gender differences. For example, women should not always serve the food and clean up afterwards and men should not always move boxes and furniture.

Recognize but Do Not Emphasize

Senior managers should not point out gender differences. They should not suggest, for example, that only a woman manager should have responsibility for the organization's child care center simply because she is a woman. Men and women should attempt to view each other as absolute equals within the workplace. This may require submerging many well-developed stereotypes.

The same concept holds true for women in senior management positions. Such "humorous" decorations as the poster that reads "It takes two men to do a woman's job" are not appropriate for the executive suite. In recent years many such slogans have arisen in the workplace. Women must work not to allow this "female supremacist" mentality to surface in their relationships, just as men must eliminate their inappropriate male biases.

Is this describing a world in which sexual differences are not noticed? Perhaps. The logic behind these suggestions is that by minimizing how often gender is a noticeable factor in the business setting, everyone can more appropriately focus on the work at hand.

Avoid Stereotyped Office Decor

Both men and women managers should avoid gender stereotypes in office decor. Male executives who display trophies and other sports paraphernalia run the risk of sending the message that they are not focused on business. For example, one hospital vice president had numerous golf-oriented pictures, signed scorecards, and trophies in his office. Some employees commented that this individual's main focus in life was not his work but his golf game. Executive women who make their offices too homelike may seem not to be focused on business. A female senior executive in a midwestern hospital had a large number of stuffed animals in her office. Although she was quite creative and successful in her position, the toys in her office caused others to wonder about her seriousness and her abilities. These suggestions are not absolute rules. It is necessary to use perspective in addressing issues of office decor. The choices in decor made by these executives might have been viewed differently had they worked in a sports medicine clinic or a children's hospital.

There Is No Such Thing as a Man's or a Woman's Job

Male managers should be considerate of what they ask peer female managers to do when working on teams and when sharing responsibilities. They must give serious consideration to whether or not their requests and expectations reflect gender biases or stereotypes, and they should avoid making requests based on unnecessary or outdated assumptions. One simple but excellent example is the expectation that female managers always handle the coffee chores or take minutes at meetings. Most men are as equipped to pour coffee or take minutes as women are, just as most women are capable of participating in moving boxes of office supplies.

Be Courteous to Members of the Opposite Sex

Managers, male and female, should be polite and not expect to follow a code of chivalry. Society today accepts using common sense when it comes to courtesy. For example, the first person reaching a door should hold it for the others.

Traditional handshaking causes a great deal of question in the workplace. Should a man offer his hand to a woman or wait for a woman to offer hers? The best rule of thumb is to always shake hands when appropriate, regardless of the who reaches out first. Women should offer their hands the same as a man would, and their handshake should be firm.

Avoid Sexual Stereotypes

Beware of gender stereotypes regarding behaviors such as aggressiveness and assertiveness. Aggressiveness is behavior meant to serve oneself and is not gender-specific. Assertiveness refers to the ability to speak for oneself while continuing to show respect for the other person. Often, women are labeled as aggressive when they actually are being what would be called assertive in a man. The problem here is in part a semantic one involving the labeling of the sexes based on an outmoded set of stereotypes. Women may be described as pushy or obstinate if they are assertive or as weak or pushovers if they are quiet. In fact, many problems between men and women are caused by the choice of words. Sexist language does not reflect well on any senior manager.

Appearance Counts

Senior managers and executives should be careful to maintain a gender-appropriate appearance. Prejudice will typically mount against executive women who look too masculine or executive men who look too feminine.

Participating in Professional Women's Groups

Women executives should feel free to participate in professional women's groups, but they must avoid joining groups that are not focused primarily on professional growth. Professional groups can help women grow and develop in their careers, build networks, and find mentors. On the other hand, taking this participation too far could keep women out of the mainstream and continue emphasizing gender-based differences. They should use judgment to prevent any interference with their work responsibilities. As a parallel, executive men who become too heavily involved in organizations that are exclusively male are continuing to promulgate the sexist differences that have no place in the senior management environment.

Working Parents

In the past, most discussions regarding working parents were focused on and directed toward women because traditionally women have been the principal caregivers. However, with men becoming increasingly involved in childcare and with the increasing number of employer-based childcare centers, children's issues have become a common concern in the workplace. Executives, whether male or female, should remember that they may sometimes be called upon—either by society, by their organization, or by their own dedication to their work—to place their jobs ahead of their families. The pressure to "do it all" may escalate as they take on the higher levels of pay and greater responsibility inherent in senior-level health care positions. Perhaps the best guideline is for senior managers and executives to work hard to ensure that childcare and other family responsibilities do not interfere with the day-to-day necessities of work. This may mean some sacrifice, but it is part of what is expected of executives. At the same time, executives should not underestimate the importance of fulfilling their personal responsibilities and taking time out for family and friends.

Summary

This chapter is based on the concept that in the workplace there should be no differences in the treatment of men and women. Although society still operates with a double standard, senior managers and executives should try to create a workplace that is as gender-neutral as possible. The protocols suggest that one should not even notice whether another person is male or female. Senior managers and executives trying to develop sensitivity to off-limits behavior and minimize behaviors and actions that might damage their career and effectiveness will find that they can enhance their careers by ignoring sexual differences.

This chapter has intentionally avoided any discussion of the alleged strengths and weaknesses of men and women in management. Readers can avail themselves of the excellent resources on this subject. Two recommended books are *Women and Men in Management* by Gary N. Powell and *Gender Stereotypes: Traditions and Alternatives* by Susan A. Basow.[1]

Consider the delicate balance in this chapter. The protocols try to avoid actions that will perpetuate sexual stereotypes and make it more difficult for women to succeed in the business world. Women should feel free to participate fully in executive life, but they should continue to be aware of possible misperceptions that such participation can create. With the new preponderance of women in the workplace, neither sex can go blindly into any kind of activity without considering the consequences or reaction of others. This is the message of the entire book and the central theme of this chapter.

Note

1. G. N. Powell, *Women and Men in Management* (Newbury Park, CA: Sage Publications, 1988); S. A. Basow, *Gender Stereotypes: Traditions and Alternatives* (Pacific Grove, CA: Brooks/Cole Publishing, 1986).

20

PUTTING IT ALL TOGETHER:
CHANGING FOR THE BETTER

How can senior managers and executives put these protocols into action? How can they break old habits?

This chapter will help to bridge the gap between the seminar and the management office, between the recognition of problems outlined in this and other books and the corresponding change in actions.

The message behind the protocols is that if senior managers and executives practice appropriate behavior, then they will become better leaders and thus will lead better organizations. Ultimately, this should make them more successful.

Readers might expect this chapter to contain testimonials from numerous health care executives who have practiced these appropriate behaviors and attribute their successes to them and examples of senior managers who have experienced job loss and career failure because of mistakes in these areas. However, this chapter has neither testimonials nor cautionary tales. All readers know of people who have violated practically every precept and principle in this book (and more) and have and continue to be quite successful (by most standards). Every example of appropriate and inappropriate behavior given in this book is true. Many others could be cited. Many of the people in the examples of "inappropriate behavior" are considered quite successful.

By following the protocols in this book senior managers will not *guarantee* their success nor their automatic progress to increasingly higher positions. But practicing the protocols will assist them in their executive careers. Knowledge and application of these standards will assist any aspiring young manager in getting along better with peers, subordinates, and more senior executives. Even very senior executives can benefit from measuring their behavior against some appropriate standard.

Do Not Jump to Conclusions

There are several general caveats for the readers of this book. First, there is always a certain amount of luck involved in executive growth. Other than the usual hard work and dedication, some good fortune is helpful along the way. Some would argue that luck is self-made in that the lucky person works hard to ensure that there are fortuitous breaks that assist in executive development.

The second caveat is embodied in the concept of a protocol (as outlined in this book). Because they are presented in a somewhat strict prescriptive fashion, there may be a tendency for some readers to view each protocol as though it is an absolute rule. In fact, however, there may exist at certain times and in certain places exceptions to practically all of the book's protocols. Many of the protocols may not always fit every situation. Most achievement-oriented managers are adaptable, flexible, have good judgment, and have a sense of the appropriate. Senior managers who view the world simplistically and require absolutes will have difficulties in dealing with many issues other than executive behavior.

There are some occasions when some eccentric behavior may be positive. Sameness is not always the correct approach to leadership. Often some differences will help senior managers set themselves apart and will enhance their leadership ability.

Finally, readers should understand the central message of this book. It has not been the intent to present rules and regulations by which aspiring senior managers and successful executives must live. The suggestions in this book should not be viewed as complete and conclusive guidelines for health care managers. Rather, the book is meant to make health care managers aware of the fourth factor of executive success and get them to begin to focus on issues other than mission and margin. It is hoped that many can become even more successful as a result.

How to Improve

The first step to improvement in any situation is to understand the issues. In the case of protocols for executive behavior, it requires a full understanding of oneself. Whether it is called self-perception, self-image, self-awareness, or self-concept, it nonetheless requires a full and complete knowledge of one's thoughts, ideals, rationales for behavior, and tendencies for action.

Senior managers and executives who truly know what and why they think, feel, and believe and understand the grounds for their behavior and actions have already taken a major step toward improvement.

Of course, it is virtually impossible to have a complete picture of oneself. However, the Johari Window is an excellent tool for self-analysis. The Johari Window describes four areas of behavior, beliefs, and actions for any individual. These four areas are divided into four "windowpanes." The first windowpane includes those areas that both an individual and others know. The second windowpane describes that which is known by the individual but is falsified so that others see something different (a facade). The third windowpane is that area which is known by others but not by the individual (the individual's blind spot). The fourth windowpane is the area that is not known by anyone.

This book involves increasing the size of the first windowpane—that which is visible and known to both the individual and others. As this is done, one's natural character begins to guide behavior in appropriate directions. Senior managers and executives begin to become genuine leaders, without pretense.

People are complex beings with myriad thoughts and perceptions. How much we know about ourselves in a dynamic world (the first windowpane) is constantly changing. The world and the way in which we see it change so quickly that it is difficult to fully categorize our approaches to it. We change, the world changes, and others within the world change.

As we fulfill our many different roles in life, we see ourselves in different lights. A chief executive may at the same time be a spouse, a parent, a son, a brother, a church leader, a neighbor, and a friend. Each one of these roles is different and demands different expectations. For example, a female executive may be both a stern governing manager and a loving, caring mother. For some, these two roles may be so conflicting that the self-perception cannot be fixed. Protocols may at times help executives work through these conflicts.

Self-Understanding

Understanding oneself is an ongoing process that is best accomplished in two ways. First, the senior manager needs another person who can serve as a mirror to reflect his or her reality. The other person must be knowledgeable enough to understand the situations faced by senior managers and articulate enough to explain what he or she is observing.

A mentor can fulfill this role. A mentor must be someone who can establish an atmosphere of trust as well as someone who ideally has experienced many, if not all, of the experiences that the person who seeks guidance is facing and will face. The word *mentor* comes from Greek mythology; Mentor was a friend of Odysseus whom Odysseus put in charge of his son. The idea of mentorship is one that has come of age in health care and has become more formalized of late.

Peers can also help others see and understand themselves. Unfortunately, with the degree of competitiveness within most organizations, it can be risky to utilize peers for this function. However, there are others who can serve in this capacity. Alumni of graduate programs are often familiar enough with a senior manager to serve as a rebound critic. Other business acquaintances in other fields can also be helpful.

The second way in which senior managers can develop a better understanding of self is through self-examination. In this situation, one evaluates oneself against some preestablished criteria. Taking graduate-level courses is one way to help in this endeavor. Continuing education programs, seminars, and workshops are other ways to better understand oneself. A number of professional societies offer self-assessment programs.

Self-Management

Prior to making any attempts at self-improvement, individuals must feel some need to improve. Organizational behavior literature talks about the concept of self-management and the antecedents of this activity. Simply put, the readers of this book must have some self-motivation to change their behaviors. They must fear job loss or inability to gain a promotion, or some other disruption in their career paths. Senior managers must believe that there are better and easier ways to lead their managerial lives. There must be some belief that what one is doing is having negative outcomes. Furthermore, there must be a conviction that practicing all or some of the protocols in this book will enhance one's chances for keeping a job, gaining a promotion, or moving to a higher position.

In *Helping People Change: A Textbook of Methods,* Frederic H. Kanfer talks about self-management by suggesting that it begins with a disruption in a person's routine.[1] The disruption can be major—such as job loss— or minor. A simple New Year's resolution to improve one's management style can be motivation enough. Kanfer then goes on to describe a three step process:

Stage 1. Self-monitoring
           To understand what one is doing.

Stage 2. Self-evaluation
    To understand of what one should do.

Stage 3. Self-reinforcement
    To understand that what one is doing is correct.

To sum up, before senior managers and executives can improve, they must be convinced that there is some good reason to change. Whether a negative or positive motivator, the feeling of need must be present and long-lasting enough to last through the monitoring, evaluation, and correction levels. There must be some sense of personal and professional urgency for senior managers.

Developing New Patterns

Here are some final protocol suggestions that may help readers hoping to break old behavior patterns and develop new ones.

Continue Studying Health Care

Senior managers must be devoted to the continuing study of health care management. They should identify successful leaders and catalog their characteristics to better study what makes them successful. They should then compare their behavior to these examples.

Study Those Who Fail

On the other side of the coin, senior managers should find out as much as possible about those who lose their jobs. They should attempt to identify any common threads that fit within the discussion of the fourth factor of executive success as identified within this book.

Expand the Network

Senior managers should take every opportunity to network with other health care executives. They should compare notes about successes and failures and talk openly about inadequacies and mistakes.

Continue One's General Education

This is different from learning more about the health care field in particular. This protocol suggests that senior managers and executives should commit to lifelong continuing education. This can be done through programs offered by the American College of Healthcare Executives or other professional organizations as well as by taking the time to read professional journals.

Become a Mentor

Senior managers and executives who have not served as mentors to others will be surprised at the valuable lessons they learn as they are challenged and questioned about what they do and why they do it. Serving as a mentor offers an opportunity to grow and develop.

Leave the Ego in the Closet

Perhaps the biggest stumbling block in changing one's behavior is one's ego. To get to many senior management positions today, a person must often develop a tough, strong personality. A high level of self-confidence is necessary to set and achieve lofty goals and make difficult decisions. As a result, many managers who rise within organizations have lost the ability to be humble and to accept that they may be wrong at times.

Executives should listen to the signs and signals around them. If people who work with and for them are willing to make specific suggestions about how they can improve, senior managers should listen to their advice. The less senior managers listen to their peers, superiors, and subordinates, the fewer opportunities they will have to receive counsel and the more isolated they will become. It is acceptable and appropriate to concede that one is imperfect and has a desire and willingness to improve.

Concluding Remarks

The messages of this book are simple:

1. All senior managers and executives have blind spots. These increase in number the higher in an organization the person is.

2. Many of these blind spots involve seemingly simple, basic issues, ones that many would not consider serious, but that can add up to an overall diminution in success and effectiveness.

3. Many executives have lost their jobs because of these issues, and amazingly, have not been at all aware of the problems before it was too late to change.

4. There are appropriate and inappropriate behaviors in the workplace. Effective senior managers and executives learn this and try to anticipate the effect their actions and behavior will have on others

and focus on always behaving appropriately. This sense of the appropriate is a crucial component of executive success.

5. As this sense of the appropriate becomes part of the character of senior managers and executives, they will generally find themselves becoming increasingly successful and will become better role models for others in the field.

Note

1. F. H. Kanfer, *Helping People Change: A Textbook of Methods*, 4th ed. (Needham Heights, MA: Allyn and Bacon Publishing, 1991), 145–46.

About the Author

Carson F. Dye, M.B.A., received his bachelor's degree from Marietta College in 1974 and his M.B.A. from Xavier University in 1977. From 1974 to 1982, he held senior human resources positions at Clermont Mercy Hospital and Children's Hospital Medical Center in Cincinnati, Ohio. From 1982 to 1990, he was administrator of human resources for The Ohio State University Hospitals. In 1990, he assumed his current position of vice president of human resources for St. Vincent Medical Center in Toledo, Ohio.

Currently, he is also an adjunct faculty member in the Division of Hospital and Health Services Administration at The Ohio State University. He has also held faculty appointments at the University of Cincinnati, teaching labor law and management, and at Xavier University, teaching in the graduate program in hospital administration.

Mr. Dye has published several articles on human resources and has worked extensively in management development and organizational design. He has taught more than 5,000 hospital and health care first-line supervisors and department heads in various leadership development areas.

Along with his interest in executive protocols, he has particular expertise in managerial ethics, values-based leadership, and rebuilding faltering human resources programs.

Currently, Mr. Dye, along with Dr. Stephen Strasser, conducts ongoing national seminars for the American College of Healthcare Executives in human resources management. A member of the College, he is also active in several other managerial and professional organizations.